FASHIONS OF THE ROARING 1920S

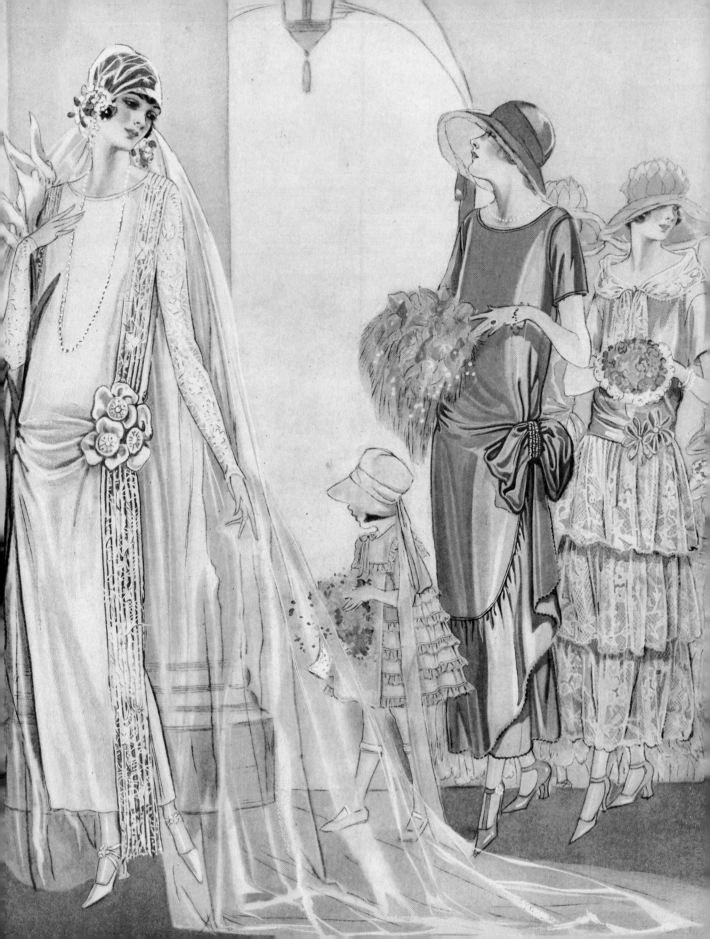

FASHIONS

of the
Roaring
'20s

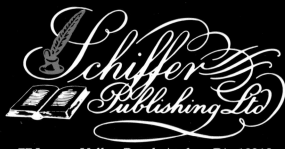

77 Lower Valley Road, Atglen, PA 19310

ACKNOWLEDGMENTS

I am indebted to the following individuals:

My husband Paul...for his patience and support.

Roseann Ettinger...for inspiring me to write and holding my hand through the various stages.

Suzanjoy M. Checksfield...for sharing with me her wealth of knowledge about vintage jewelry and allowing me to photograph so many of her special treasures.

Joan Ligon...for her assistance with French terms and pronunciations.

Rose and Paul Jamieson and Ellis Grumer for their enthusiasm and patience during the numerous photography sessions of their lovely jewelry and related objects from the 1920s.

Mary Anne Faust...for sharing her vintage clothing experitise and for helping with the price guide.

My brother Robbie Pascoe...for his computer assistance.

I would also like to thank the people of the following institutions:

Allentown Public Library, Allentown, Pa.

Cedar Crest College Alumni Museum, Cedar Crest College, Allentown, Pa.

Costume Library, Costume Institute, Metropolitan Museum of Art, New York, NY.

Dan's Camera City, Allentown, Pa.

East Stroudsburg University, East Stroudsburg, Pa.

Kemerer Museum of Decorative Arts, Bethlehem, Pa.

Lehigh County Historical Society, Allentown, Pa.

Whiting & Davis Company Handbag Museum, Attleboro Falls, Ma.

To the memory of my mother-in-law, the late Margaretha J. Laubner, who, in 1981, encouraged me to begin collecting vintage clothing and accessories by presenting me with many old dresses, beaded bags, and eyeglasses.

To my own mother, Elizabeth Pascoe Whitfield, who has so generously given her time and talents over the past years to accompany me on the lecture circuit and beautifully mend the many garments I have placed in her care.

Library of Congress Cataloging-in-Publication Data

Laubner, Ellie.
  Fashions of the Roaring '20s / Ellie Laubner.
      p. cm.
  Includes bibliographical references and index.
  ISBN 0-7643-0017-2 (pbk.)
  1. Costume--United States--History--20th century. 2. Fashion--United States--History--20th century. I. Title.
GT615.L38 1996
391'.00973'09042--dc20   96-15436
                                     CIP

Printed in Hong Kong
ISBN: 0-7643-0017-2

Published by Schiffer Publishing Ltd.
77 Lower Valley Road
Atglen, PA 19310
Please write for a free catalog.
This book may be purchased from the publisher.
Please include $2.95 for shipping.
Try your bookstore first.

Frontispiece: Bride—long slender gown accented with silk flowers at the dropped waist, veil gathered over head with clusters of blossoms over each ear, long stemmed Calla lillies. / Flower girl—poke bonnet and ruffled dress. / Attendants— wide brim hats, strapy shoes (one shoe button cover). *Delineator, 4/24.*

CONTENTS

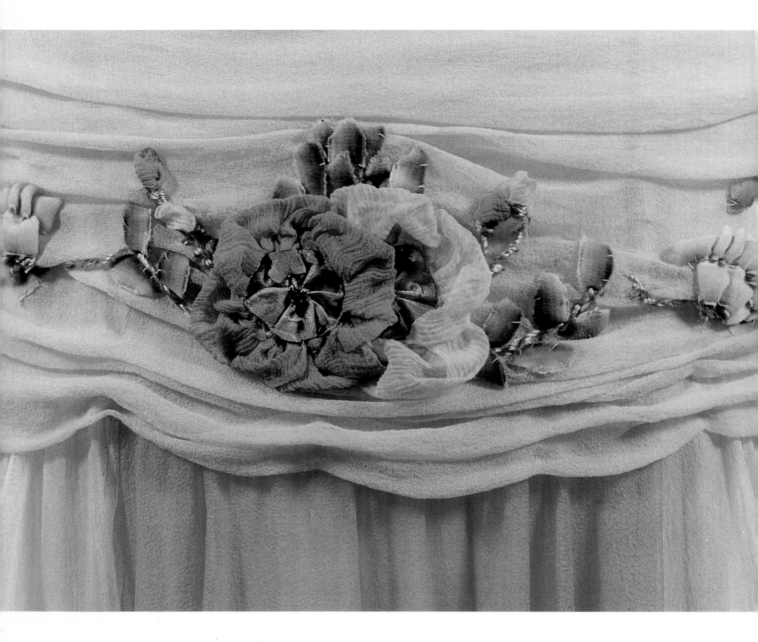

Detail from yellow and orange flapper dress, c. 1925-1929.

INTRODUCTION

Fashion trends have simultaneously shaped and been influenced by history and current events. Therefore, when we look at the predominant styles of any given period, what we are seeing are reflections of the morals, customs, etiquette, new technology, and the mood of that period. There is also a strong correlation between fashion and the decorative arts, architecture, and interior design of an era. Once you are able to "read" them, fashions from the past can provide clues to the social and cultural history of the period in which they were worn. Those studying the history of costume will find it more interesting and easier to understand if they can relate the styles of a period to the events which influenced them.

France has been the leader of fashion since the days of Louis XIV, so consequently many fashion terms are in the French language. In order to accommodate for this, I have included the definitions and pronunciations of French words in the glossary located at the end of the book.

The objects pictured on the following pages chronicle this period of dramatic change. They epitomize the heyday of the flapper and her emancipation in our society.

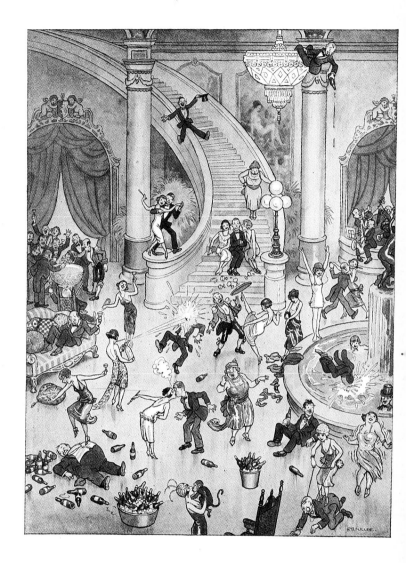

Cartoon by R. B. Fuller picturing a wild 1920s party which graphically illustrates the effects of prohibition. *Judge,* 3/28/25.

CHAPTER 1:

HISTORICAL BACKGROUND OF THE 1920S

The morals, customs, and mood of the 1920s were a drastic departure from those of the two preceding decades. During the First World War, women were called upon to fill the jobs that the men left behind. There was no time for mincing steps in restricting "hobble skirts"! Shorter, wider, more practical skirts were designed for the assertive independent women who were now earning substantial wages for their war time work.

At the end of the war, Americans were anxious to "return to normalcy." This was impossible, however, since the war had permanently changed the world. Women were unwilling to return to the confining clothing of earlier decades, or submit to the limitations these clothes represented. They proved they could handle responsibility, and in 1920 they were finally granted the right to vote.

The war created a great shortage of young men, which meant that many young women would have to become financially independent. Practical clothing was needed for those entering the male dominated occupations gradually opening up to women.

In 1919, Congress enacted the 18th Amendment which prohibited the sale of alcoholic beverages. Prohibition was meant to eliminate the alcohol problem in the United States, but unfortunately it only made matters worse. It was impossible to enforce this new law and mobsters soon began "rum running." Many people distilled their own "hooch" in homemade stills or bath tubs, thus the expression "bathtub gin." Others viewed illegal drinking as a challenging pastime and devised ingenious ways to conceal alcohol in their clothing or accessories.

Many fashionable whites frequented clandestine night clubs called "speakeasies" in the black neighborhoods of New York's Harlem. Here they drank "bootleg" whiskey, danced, and listened to black singers like Billy Holiday and musicians like Louis Armstrong and Duke Ellington perform a new style of music called Jazz.

New energetic dances like the Charleston, the Shimmy, and the Blackbottom became exercises in perpetual motion and were soon universally popular. Short dresses and shoes with straps were a reflection of the flapper's need for clothing which allowed for freedom of rapid movement. Fringed evening dresses, tasseled necklaces, and pendant earrings swished and swayed, accentuating the frenzied beat.

According to the authors of the Time/Life series *This Fabulous Century: 1920-1930*, "The '20s were an exciting—and perhaps a frightening—time to be young. It was the era of the First Youth Rebellion. Once boys tried to be paragons of gallantry, industry and idealism; girls had aspired to seem modest and maidenly. Now all that had changed."

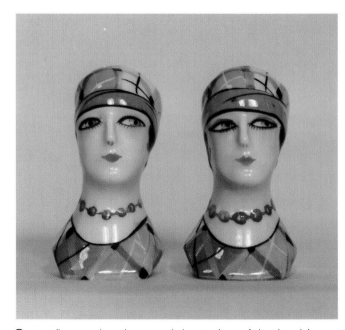

Ceramic flapper salt and pepper shakers in three of the decade's most popular colors: sunset orange, maize, and French blue. Marked: Japan. *Courtesy of Margaretha J. Laubner.*

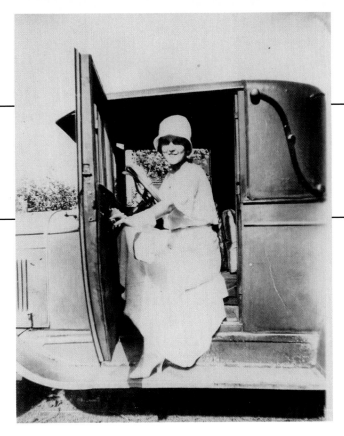

Women of the 1920s were often photographed behind the wheel of an automobile, one of the symbols of their new-found independence. *Courtesy of Rose Jamieson.*

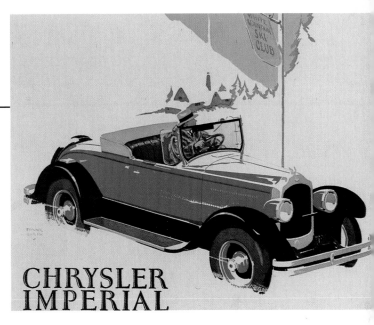

This "sheik" is the "cats meow" in his raccoon coat and sporty red roadster. *Vogue, 2/15/27.*

Many young people held the older generation responsible for the hardships of war. They appeared unconcerned with the complex problems of the world and instead preferred to spend their energies in pursuit of pleasure, excitement, and frivolity. Disregarding the disapproval of the adult generation and its old Victorian taboos, young people were "hell bent" on having a "swell" time! Teenagers became free-spirited, reckless, and daring. Cigarette smoking doubled in the 1920s. Unchaperoned couples could be seen "necking" at house parties and in parked roadsters. The fast living of the period contributed to a loosening of morals, reflected in the abbreviated skirts of the period. The sophisticated decadence of this postwar society is well documented in *The Great Gatsby* (1925) and other novels by American author F. Scott Fitzgerald.

Newly invented motion pictures were instrumental in the rapid dissemination of new styles in fashion. Clara Bow, the "It Girl" of 1920s movies ("it" meant sexual magnetism), set the standard for feminine beauty. Young girls emulated her bobbed hair, pencil thin eyebrows, and dark red "cupid's bow" lips, which became her trademark.

For hundreds of years, it had been the custom to accentuate the differences between the male and female anatomy. Now all of that had changed. As a result of the attention focused on youth, the image of the ideal feminine figure was transformed from the matronly S-bend figure of the turn of the century to the youthful, flat-chested "*garçonne*" or boyish figure of the 1920s. This androgynous look was also a reflection of women's desire to compete with men in many aspects of their lives.

The flamboyance and gaiety of the young girls was, in part, an attempt to attract the attention of the remaining male population. These giddy and uninhibited young girls, with their flippant airs, enjoyed dressing in an unconventional manner. They often wore their goulashes (Arctic boots) with the buckles unfastened so that they "flap-flapped" as they walked, thus the name "flappers."

The 1920s cartoonist, John Held, Jr., cleverly recorded the frolicsome antics of flappers and their beaus (sometimes referred to as "Held's Hellions") on the pages of *Life* and *New Yorker* magazines. His humorous cartoons captured the essence of this outrageous period in our nation's history.

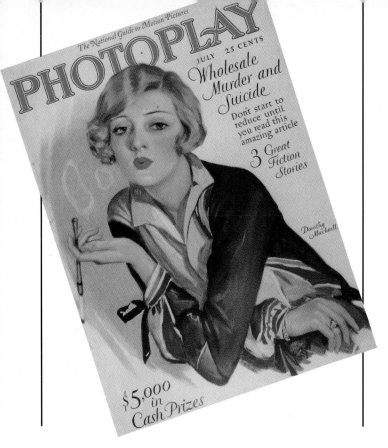

Flapper with cigarette holder, nonchalantly blowing smoke rings. *Photoplay.*

In 1925, the *Parisian Exposition International des Arts Décoratifs et Industriels Modernes,* an international exhibition of modern decorative arts, introduced to the world a new form of art which would later be called "Art Deco." This exhibition was a milestone in art history, as it was the first time that an exhibition of such magnitude was organized for the presentation of decorative art objects (as opposed to fine arts).

In stark contrast to the free flowing sentimental lines of Art Nouveau, the new Art Deco style was characterized by hard-edged geometric shapes, parallel lines, concentric circles, step patterns, sunbursts (a symbol of optimism), and waterfalls or fountains. Traditional motifs such as flowers and leaves were portrayed in a stylized fashion; i.e. the "Deco rose," which became a symbol of the Art Deco movement. Not only were geometric designs used in the ornamentation of garments and accessories, but the entire ideal feminine figure resembled a large rectangle. Art Deco was actually an eclectic synthesis of many forces including the elements of several modern art movements, as well as motifs and materials from several ancient civilizations. It incorporated clean lines from Purism, geometric interpretation and stylization from Cubism, and dynamic color combinations such as black with white, red, or green from Fauvism. It also assimilated bright colors and sumptuous fabrics from the Middle East; materials such as jade, carnelian, ivory, and lacquer from China; and geometric motifs and step patterns from the American Indian and Aztec civilizations. Even the bold *sans-serif* letters of Art Deco alphabets reflected the geometric quality of this new art movement.

Another influence on Art Deco began with the discovery of King Tutankhamen's tomb in 1922, which triggered an explosion of Egyptian style in all forms of decorative art. Scarabs, mummies, Pharaohs, papyrus, lotus blossoms, serpents, and hieroglyphics were incorporated in jewelry and fabric design with an Egyptian flair.

Art Deco jewelry, vanity cases, and smoking accessories featured futuristic industrial materials such as bakelite, chrome, and aluminum. A new "machine esthetics" developed as machines became more involved in the world of decorative arts. Engine-turnings (machine engravings) were a popular form of industrial ornamentation frequently used to embellish decorative art objects of the 1920s-30s. Machines could engrave the intricate designs in a fraction of the time required by the hand engraver.

Newer and faster modes of transportation inspired a fascination with speed, and streamlined designs began to emerge in architecture, home furnishings, textiles, and jewelry. The swift leaping gazelle motif was a common symbol of this new accelerated society.

The "It Girl" Clara Bow with a wavy bob, pencil-thin arched eyebrows, and bright red "cupid's bow" lips. *The Silent Hostess,* 1929. *Courtesy of Suzanjoy M. Checksfield.*

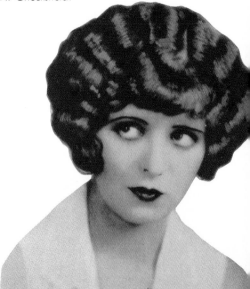

Industry boomed in the 1920s. Prices fell while wages climbed steadily upward. For those who found themselves in need of cash, an easy "deferred payment plan" could be arranged. This was a time of ostentation and conspicuous consumption (which makes this period ideal for the collector).

Through advancements in modern technology, the simple tubular dresses of the 1920s could be efficiently mass produced, providing inexpensive yet stylish ready-made fashions for working-class women. A new standardized sizing system facilitated the sale of ready-to-wear clothing. Local and national store chains were established which increased purchasing power and helped to lower the prices of consumer goods.

A modern synthetic fiber called "rayon" became a popular inexpensive substitute for silk. The use of "automatic slide fasteners" (zippers) for luggage, boots, and little girls' leggings began in the late 1920s. (They would not be used for garments until the early 1930s.)

The most influential fashion designer of the 1920s was French *couturiere* Gabrielle "Coco" Chanel who opened her couture house in 1914. She is considered by many to be the "creator of the modern woman." She seemed to know what women needed, even before they did, and her slender boyish figure made her an excellent model for her own creations. Chanel felt that traditional clothes for women were too confining and unsuited for the active women of the twenties. She was a pioneer in adapting men's fashions, such as the cardigan sweater and the blazer, into wearable casual clothes for women. Her bell-bottom beach pajamas were all the rage in the late 1920s and early 1930s. She pioneered the use of lowly wool jersey for suits and for her "little black dress" with white collar and cuffs. For daytime she favored the use of black, white, beige, and red (colors also employed by the creators of Art Deco jewelry.)

Always a trend setter, she was one of the first to "bob" her hair, smoke cigarettes, and display a sun tan, which until the 1920s was considered vulgar.

In 1922, she launched a new perfume which she simply called "Chanel No 5." She designed and promoted her "illusion jewelry" (costume jewelry) which incorporated gold chains with large imitation gem stones and synthetic pearls. Chanel is best remembered for her classic suit featuring a collarless boxy jacket with contrasting braided trim and a straight skirt. Simplicity and understated elegance were the hallmarks of all of her designs.

A feeling of optimism enticed millions of people to buy shares of stock on speculation. This eventually lead to the stock market crash of 1929, which caused many people to lose their fortunes overnight. The crash put an end to the wild and reckless spirit of the 1920s and brought the decade to an abrupt and sobering conclusion.

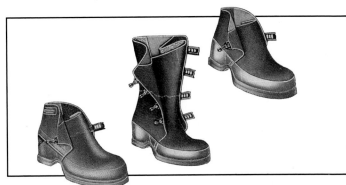

Galoshes like those worn by flappers. Montgomery Ward, 1920-21.

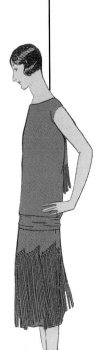

Flapper with flat-chested *garçonne* figure, modeling a tubular frock trimmed with silk fringe. *Vogue, 6/1/26. Courtesy of Richard Groman.*

Machine-embroidered trim featuring stylized Deco roses. *Courtesy of Suzanjoy M. Checksfield.*

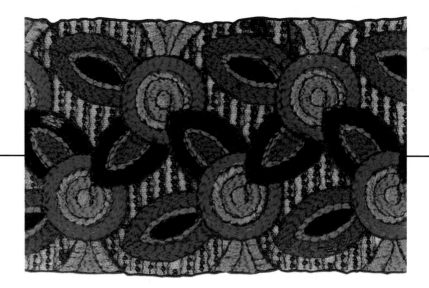

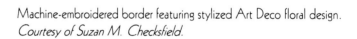

Machine-embroidered border featuring stylized Art Deco floral design. *Courtesy of Suzan M. Checksfield.*

Fashion drawing demonstrating the geometric quality of the 1920s ideal figure.

Art Deco inspired afternoon frock by Lucile of Paris. The geometric lines are accentuated by the use of graduated tones of gray. *McCall's,* 2/27.

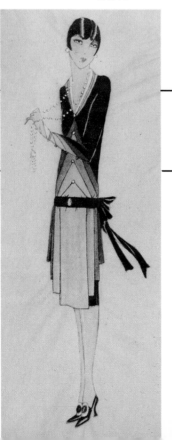

Evening gown featuring a sash with Egyptian-style scarab ornament. *Delineator,* 1923.

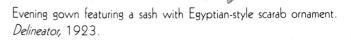

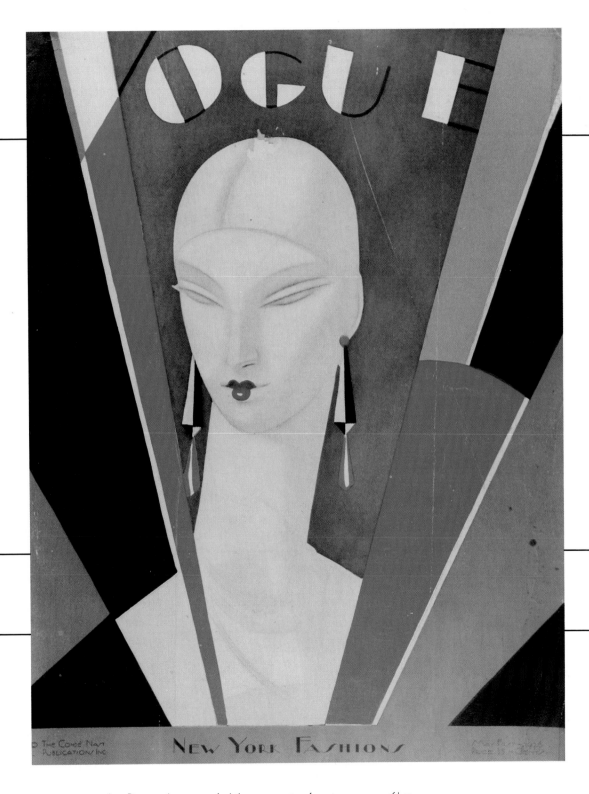

Art Deco-style cover of *Vogue* magazine featuring *sans-serif* letters, bold geometric shapes, and typical dynamic color scheme which includes red, black, and white, 5/1/26. *Courtesy of Richard Groman.*

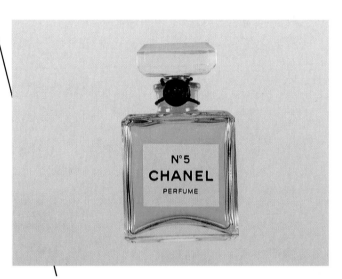

Chanel No 5 perfume in its simple, uncluttered Art Deco-style bottle.

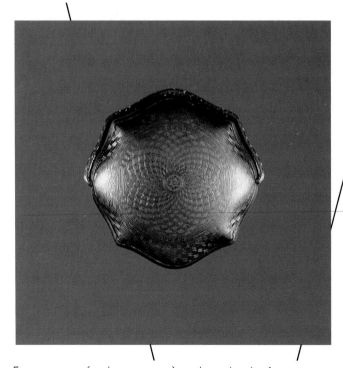

Engine-turnings (machine engraving) on the underside of a compact.

CHAPTER 2:
LINGERIE

The word lingerie is derived from the French word *linge* which means linen. It refers to ladies' intimate apparel which includes both undergarments and sleepwear.

UNDERGARMENTS

A study of 1920s undergarments often leads to confusion. Due to the overlapping of old and new styles, there was a large and diverse selection of garments from which a woman could choose. To further complicate matters, designers and manufacturers often selected different names for the same garment.

In general, fewer more abbreviated undergarments were being worn than in the past. At the turn of the century, a woman was expected to wear drawers, a chemise, a corset, a corset cover, and several petticoats under her heavy clothing. During the second half of the 1920s, a brassiere and "step-ins," or just a "teddy" were considered sufficient for those with a slender figure.

Undergarments were being made of thinner and more supple fabrics. Cotton undergarments made of nainsook, muslin, voile, batiste, sateen, plissé, and broadcloth were still available during the early 20s. However, the use of exquisite silks in the form of satin, pongee, shantung, crepe de chine, and glove silk became the indulgence of fashion conscious women of means.

A new inexpensive synthetic fiber called artificial silk (renamed rayon in 1924) was rapidly replacing cotton lingerie for middle-class women. It was made of cellulose which was obtained from plants. Slightly more lustrous than silk, this fiber could be knit or woven into soft fabric with good drapablity. Because of its high absorbency, rayon could be easily dyed.

Undergarments, formerly produced only in white, were now created in a wide spectrum of pastel colors. Peach, flesh, shell pink, and Nile green were the most common colors.

These dainty confections were often decorated with appliqués, embroidery, hemstitching, punchwork, pin tucking, picot edging, delicate ribbon flowers, and cream or ecru lace. Common laces used for lingerie were Val, Alençon, and Chantilly. Undergarments made of printed fabric became available during the second half of the decade.

The older built-up style shoulders were replaced by narrow straps made of (non-adjustable) silk ribbon or self fabric. Fancy brocade and two-toned reversible ribbon (pink with pale blue selvage on one side, and blue with pink selvage on the other) were often used. Since these narrow straps had a tendency to slip off of the shoulders, a variety of fancy lingerie clips and pins were devised to support the straps, fasten undergarment straps to each other, or pin the straps to the garment.

Because of the increased attention focused on the younger generation, the ideal matronly "S-bend" silhouette of the *Belle Epoque* was replaced by a slender, more youthful figure. This figure may be characterized as a cylinder with no indication of a bust or waist, bearing more resemblance to a young boy than a woman.

Since straight was in and curves were out, new undergarments had to be devised to squash, flatten, and obliterate all traces of the feminine curve. Women selected their undergarments based upon their individual figures and the amount of flattening and reshaping they considered necessary to produce the desired figure.

BANDEAU

The low slung matronly "monobosom" so admired at the turn of the century was replaced by the flat-chested look of the 1920s. Women relied on a *bandeau* to compress and flatten the bust. This garment was also known as a bust bodice, bust confiner, or a brassiere. The *bandeau* consisted of a strip of fabric (without cups), which was fastened tightly across the bust. Silk or rayon jersey, crepe de chine, satin, or lace were used for the slender figure; while *coutil* (a firm cotton twill), *broché* (a heavy brocade), and para rubber were used for firm control of the larger figure. *Bandeaux* contained ribbon straps and a corset tab.

Towards the end of the decade, renewed admiration for a natural anatomical shape lead to the creation of a shorter "cup-form" brassiere. This brassiere was designed with gathers between the breasts to lift, separate, and provide mild shaping.

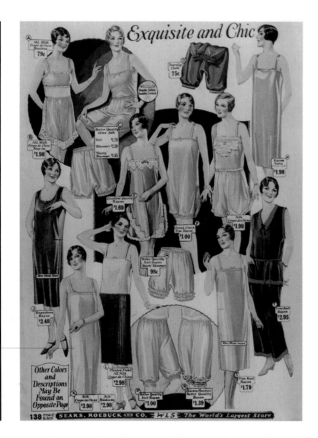

Lingerie ad: A-*bandeau*, B-step-ins, C-vest & bloomers, D, M, P, R-bloomers, E, G-teddies, F-camiknickers, H, J, K, S-slips, L-bodice skirt, T-pajamas in Deco colors, red and black. Sears, Roebuck and Co., 1928-29.

CORSET

The dropped waist was unflattering to the "pear-shaped" figure, since a horizontal line placed over wide hips only emphasizes their width. For firm control of the larger figure, the corset was still a necessity. Sometimes referred to as a girdle, this garment extended from below the breasts to mid-thigh and was designed to "eliminate unbecoming fullness in the hips and abdomen." Corsets were usually made of *coutil* or *broché* with elastic inserts for comfort. They were still heavily boned and were fastened with hooks and lacing. Four to six "hose supporters" (metal garters) were suspended from the corset on strips of elastic. The corset was worn over a vest, camiknickers, or step-in-chemise (see descriptions below). As unlikely as it may seem, there were even maternity corsets designed to give support during pregnancy.

According to Frederick Lewis Allen, the author of an informative book on the 1920s titled *Only Yesterday*, proper mothers insisted that their daughters wear girdles to dances. Many girls felt they were too restrictive for the energetic dances of the period and went directly to the ladies' room to remove them.

BANDEAU CORSET

Also referred to as a doublette, a corset brassiere, a *corselé*, or a *corselette* (also spelled corselet), the *bandeau* corset was a combination of the *bandeau* and the corset. Its long-line construction flattened unsightly bulges and provided a smooth unbroken line from bust to thigh. They were generally made of *coutil* or *broché* with four to six hose supporters.

PETTICOAT

Calf-length sateen, silk jersey, and changeable taffeta petticoats (half slips) were worn in the early years of the decade until short slender skirts rendered them obsolete. They were decorated with ruffles, tiers, and flounces.

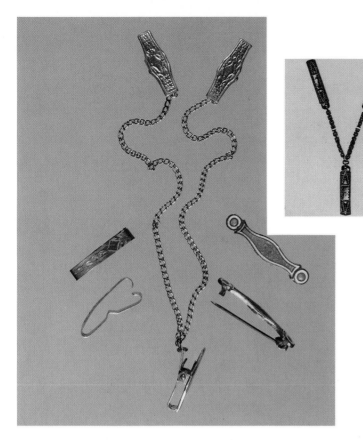

Left - Two gold-plated lingerie clips. Center - Three nickel-plated spring-loaded lingerie clips fastened together with chains. Right - Two Nile green *cloisonné* lingerie pins.

BLOOMERS

Also called knickers, these loose-fitting underpants were gathered just above the knee with elastic or knee bands. The waist was either all elastic or consisted of a pointed waist yoke in front and elastic in back. They were usually made of silk or rayon.

CAMIKNICKERS

One-piece camiknickers were a combination of the camisole and knickers. They were also known as cami-bockers, bloomer combinations, cami-combinations, chemise-knickers, teddy bloomers, or bloomer suits. Some camiknickers were constructed with elastic knee bands, while others had plackets on the sides of the legs. A convenient "drop seat" was frequently placed in the rear.

STEP-IN DRAWERS

Named for the method of putting them on, step-in-drawers, step-in-panties, step-ins, or just plain drawers were loose underpants resembling a short slightly flared skirt. The pointed waist yokes (front and back) were cut on the straight of the fabric, while the side pieces were cut on the bias, allowing the fabric to fall in graceful fluted folds.

SLIP

The tubular slip had a straight drawstring top with self fabric, lace, or ribbon straps. Pleats or gathers were placed over each hip for ease of fit and freedom of movement. Slips with deep shadow-proof hems (hip to knee) were worn as a necessity under the sheer silk chiffon dresses of the late twenties. Many sheer dresses contained their own matching slips.

STEP-IN-CHEMISE

Also known as a step-in-combination, an envelope chemise and a teddy, the step-in-chemise was a combination of the chemise (or vest) and step-in-drawers. Made of crepe de chine or rayon, they resembled a short tubular slip with a stitched or buttoned crotch.

CAMISOLE

In place of the old cotton corset cover with lace yoke and built-up straps, a new silk or rayon camisole emerged with a straight top and ribbon straps. It was gathered at the top with pastel ribbon and at the waist with elastic. The camisole could either be worn over, under, or in place of the *bandeau*. It was worn until the late 1920s when it was replaced by the vest.

VEST

The vest had a straight drawstring top with ribbon straps. It was generally thigh length and was worn tucked into knickers or drawers. Glove silk or rayon jersey were the common fabrics used to make this rather plain garment.

UNION SUIT

Also known as "long johns," the popular one-piece union suit had long, short, or no sleeves, and long or short legs. It buttoned up the center front and had a convenient drop seat in the rear. They were made of cotton or wool knit and were worn for warmth by both sexes and all ages.

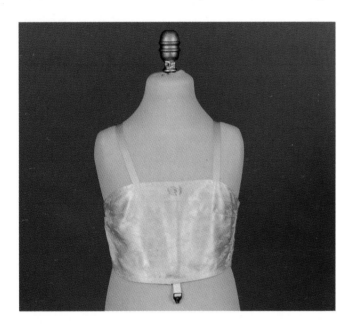

Peach *broché bandeau*—ribbon straps, ribbon rosette, corset tab. *Photo by Bradley Schaeffer.*

Pink silk satin and white lace *bandeau. Courtesy of Mary Anne Faust (Yesterday's Delights). Photo by Bradley Schaeffer.*

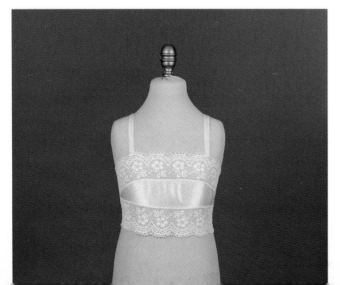

DRESS SHIELDS

Crescent-shaped dress shields, made of rubberized cloth, were worn under the arms to prevent perspiration stains.

HOSE

The colors of hose or stockings changed dramatically during the twenties. Early hose were usually limited to black, white, beige, brown, and gunmetal. As skirts became shorter, women preferred to wear more alluring pastel or flesh-toned hose. Daring young women could be seen wearing the transparent "nude look" hose which at the time was considered quite shocking! Black hose were still available but were worn primarily with black evening dresses, sportswear, or for mourning. When suntanning came into vogue, deeper flesh tones called "sunburn" and "golden tan" were offered.

Lisle Hose

Opaque lisle hose were made of inexpensive durable cotton which was often mercerized to increase the luster. Lisle hose were worn for housework, sports, and walking. They were generally made with a striped or honeycomb rib, or attractive blue and tan plaid. Some stocking styles were full length, while others were turned down below the knee to form a cuff.

Silk Hose

The preferred and also the most expensive hose were made of transparent silk. Special dance hose were made of silk chiffon with an innerfoot and garter hem of cotton lisle for strength.

Rayon Hose

Semi-transparent rayon hose resembled silk in its lustrous appearance, but cost considerably less. It was first used for stockings in 1912, and soon replaced lisle as the inexpensive alternative to silk. (Hose were also made in various blends of these fibers.)

I interviewed several former flappers who had occasion to wear hose made from both silk and rayon. They reported that silk hose were finer, softer, warmer, less baggy, quicker drying, and also had less tendency to slide down the leg than rayon hose.

It was the custom for frolicking flappers to be photographed while hiking up their skirts to show off their knees. Silk and rayon hose are often recognizable in photographs of the twenties because of their sheen.

Desirable "full fashion marks," "fashioning marks" or "fashion points" were small dots in the knit along the seam created by increasing or decreasing stitches.

Pointed "dagger" and "step-up" designs were knitted into the heels of stockings to decorate and "slenderize the ankle." Fancy silk evening hose of the late 1920s and early 1930s were embroidered in vertical arrows or patterns over the ankles called "clocks" (occasionally spelled clox in 1920s catalogs). Stockings were also decorated with lace inserts.

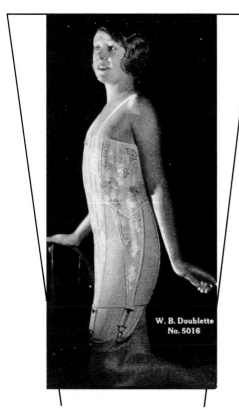

Weingarten Bros. ad for bust flattening brocaded doublette (*bandeau* corset). *Vogue*, 10/25.

GARTERS

Two types of circular garters were employed during the 1920s.

Utilitarian Garters

Utilitarian roll garters were made of round tubular elastic. They were placed over the top of the stockings which were then rolled down over them. Garters were mainly worn by young women who did not need, or did not choose to wear a confining girdle or garter belt to support their hose. Skirt lengths reached their shortest in 1925, when they ended just below the knee. Skirt hems only slightly overlapped the tops of stockings, creating a problem of how to conceal the garter hems of hose. This problem was playfully captured in many of the cartoons by John Held, Jr. Garters were also mentioned in this popular 1920s song by Ray Henderson.

Five Foot Two, Eyes of Blue

Five foot two,
Eyes of blue,
But oh! what those five feet can do,
Has anybody seen my girl?

Turned up nose,
Rolled down hose,
Flapper, yah she's one of those,
Has anybody seen my girl?

Ornamental Garters

Ornamental flat garters called "jazz garters" were worn on top of the hose, above the knee, for decorative purposes only. They were made of flat elastic covered with satin or moiré ribbon and trimmed with lace and dainty ribbon flowers. Four-piece "dance sets" consisted of a *bandeau*, stepins, and two jazz garters which flashed provocatively during the frenzied dancing of the period.

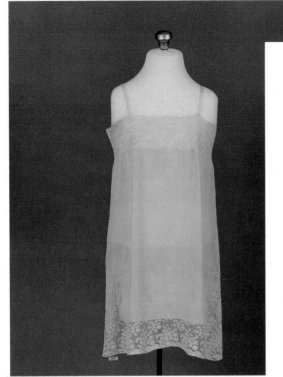

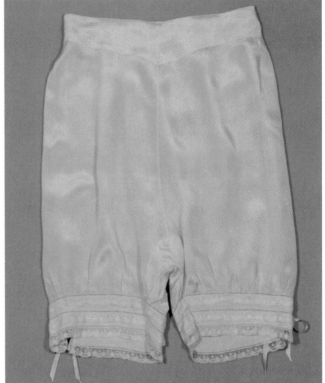

Peach silk straight-line slip with ecru lace. *Courtesy of Catherine Tobin. Photo by Bradley Schaeffer.*

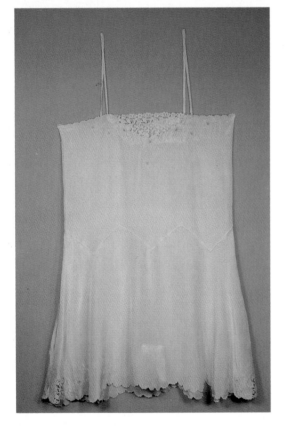

Pink silk crepe de chine bloomers—waist yoke; knee bands with val lace ruffles, hemstitching, and ribbon ties.

White silk crepe de chine teddy—embroidery, Honiton lace.

Ivory crepe de chine teddy with val lace, ribbon rosettes.

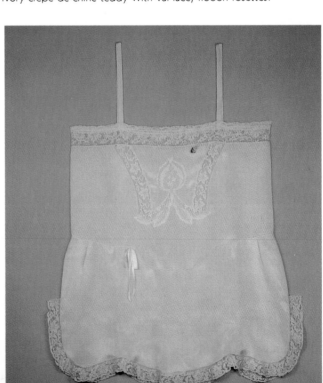

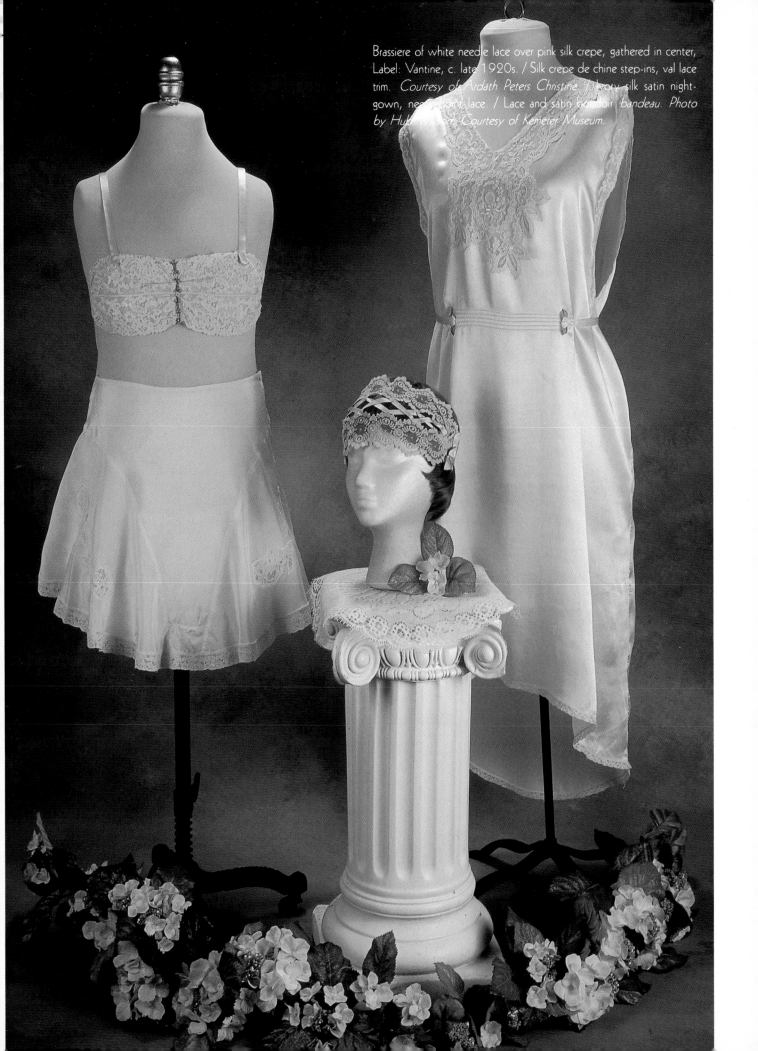

Brassiere of white needle lace over pink silk crepe, gathered in center, Label: Vantine, c. late 1920s. / Silk crepe de chine step-ins, val lace trim. *Courtesy of Ardath Peters Christine.* / Ivory silk satin nightgown, needlepoint lace. / Lace and satin boudoir bandeau. *Photo by Hub Wilson, Courtesy of Kemeter Museum.*

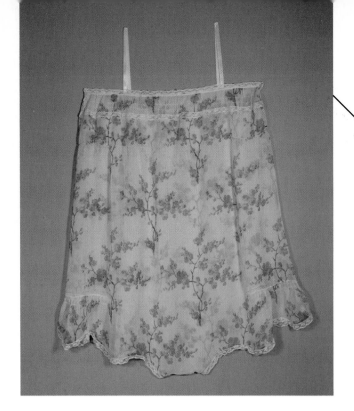

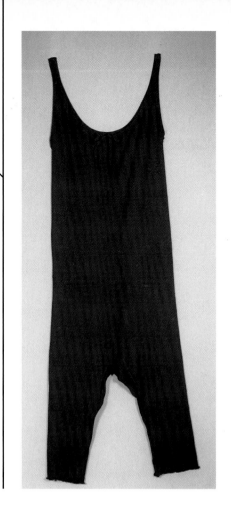

Sheer silk georgette floral-print teddy—drawstring top, val lace trim. *Courtesy of Grace Voorhees Howells.*

Plain tubular rayon knit vest—drawstring top, ribbon straps. Label: Blue Swan. *Courtesy of Cedar Crest Alumnae Museum, gift of Ellie Laubner.*

Black sleeveless cotton knit union suit—scoop neckline with drawstring, short legs. Label: The Viola. *Courtesy of Cedar Crest Alumnae Museum, gift of Ellie Laubner.*

Silk stockings in the soft shades worn during the 1920s. Far right—short red hose to be worn with roll garters, marked: Rolette. *Courtesy of Jean Weaber. Photo by Bradley Schaeffer.*

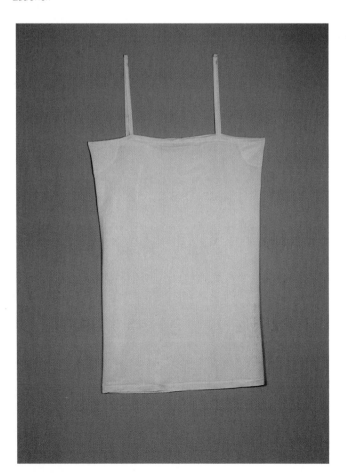

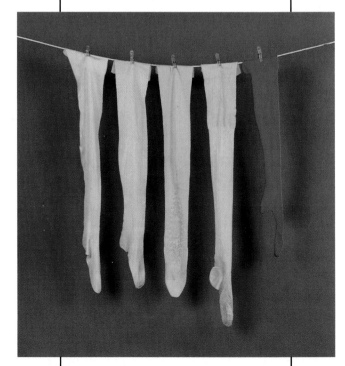

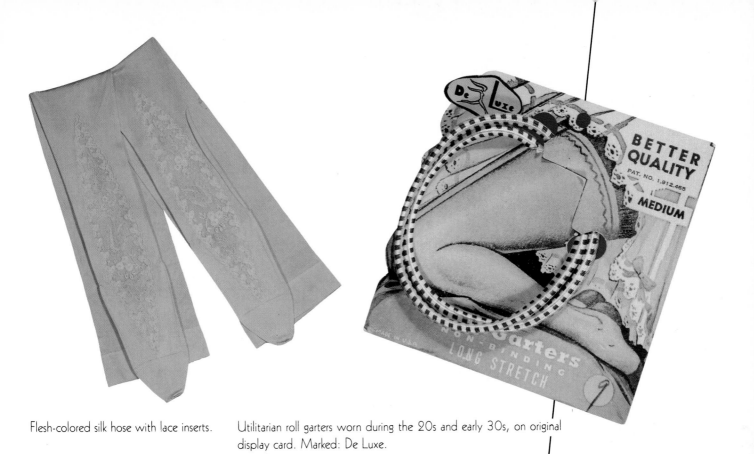

Flesh-colored silk hose with lace inserts.

Utilitarian roll garters worn during the 20s and early 30s, on original display card. Marked: De Luxe.

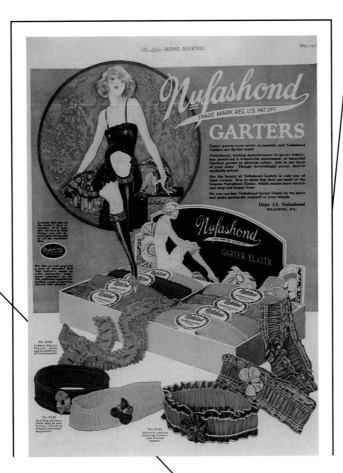

Ornamental flat garters with ribbon rosettes by Nufashund. *Ladies Home Journal*, May 1925.

SLEEPWEAR

NIGHTGOWNS

Ankle-length nightgowns, without darts, were made with a square or a V-neckline. They were offered in nainsook, voile, plissé, flannelette, rayon jersey, satin, and various silk weaves. Also available were cotton batiste nightgowns which were hand embroidered in the Philippines or Puerto Rico.

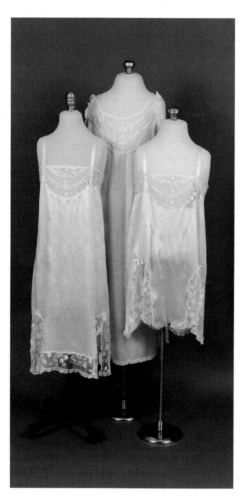

Items from bride's trousseau—slip, nightgown, and teddy of ivory silk satin, handmade appliquéd lace, 1927. *Courtesy of Kemerer Museum, gift of Lucia Gray. Photo by Bradley Schaeffer.*

Blue satin pajamas—white godets at bottom of wide-leg pants, blue and white Oriental embroidery, c. 1925-30. *Courtesy of Mary Anne Faust (Yesterday's Delights). Photo by Bradley Schaeffer.*

PAJAMAS

Pajama stems from the Hindi word "*paejama*" which means leg clothing. A fascination with exotic apparel from the East, lead to the popularization of pajamas for sleeping, lounging, or sitting on the beach. They consisted of a sleeveless V-neck tunic (with or without a sash) worn over loose-fitting wide-leg pants. Pajamas were made of silk, rayon, or cotton in solid, figured, or border print fabrics. Pastel colors were popular as well as the combination of red and black (typical Art Deco colors). By 1929, "tuck-in pajamas" were made with tops which were tucked into the pants.

COOLIE COATS

Many "pajama suits" were offered with a matching coolie coat or short Chinese-style robe featuring kimono sleeves. This handy jacket was used for lounging at home or as a cover-up at the beach.

Red cotton coolie coat—Oriental characters and floral motif. Worn in dormitory by co-ed at Wilson College, 1928-32. *Courtesy of Ethel Bishop.*

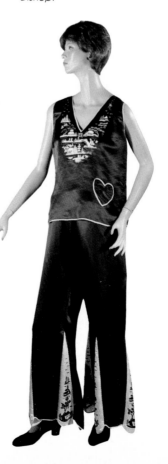
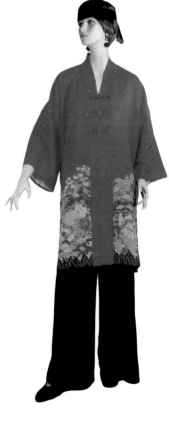

"BILLIE BURKE"

Named for Ziegfeld Follie's star Billie Burke, these one-piece pajamas resembled a loose-fitting jumpsuit. They had buttons or frogs along the center front opening, and an open crotch or drop seat for convenience. They were usually made of nainsook or flannelette with elastic at the ankles which created a short ruffle. This style was a carry-over from the teens.

twisted rayon cord girdle and satin trim. Quilted satin, terry cloth, flannel, and silk were also used for robes and were often enhanced with contrasting shawl collars, cuffs, and sashes.

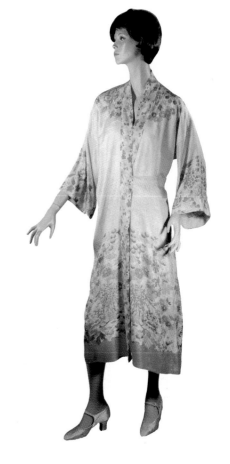

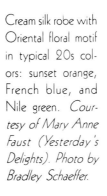

Cream silk robe with Oriental floral motif in typical 20s colors: sunset orange, French blue, and Nile green. *Courtesy of Mary Anne Faust (Yesterday's Delights). Photo by Bradley Schaeffer.*

Flannelette "Billie Burke"—ruffles at ankles; button or frog closings; trimmed with braid, hemstitching, and embroidery. Montgomery Ward, 1920-21.

ROBES

Surplice-style robes, which tied or buttoned over the right hip, were available in a myriad of fabrics. Soft snugly blanket-cloth robes, available from the Beacon and the Lawrence companies, were popular for both sexes and all ages. They were made in geometric and floral prints with a

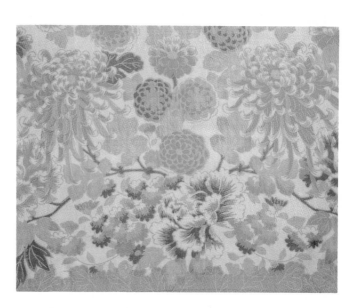

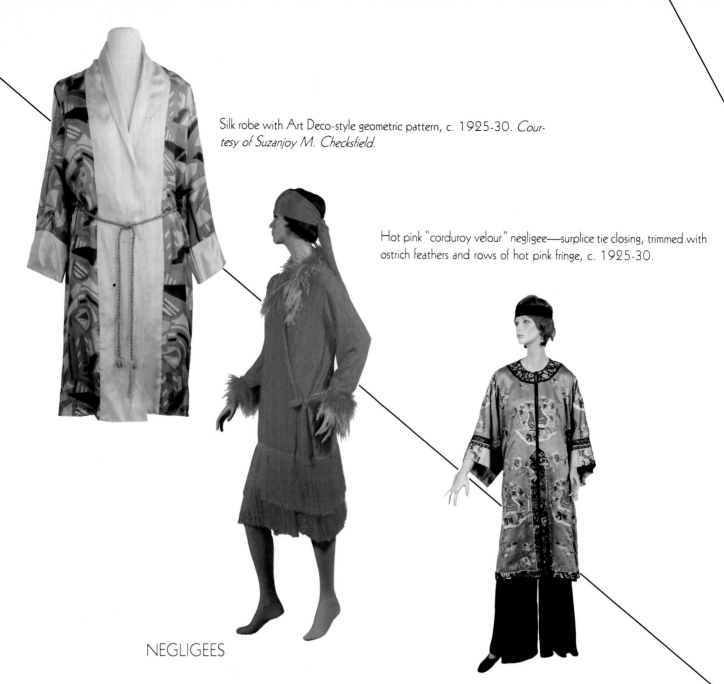

Silk robe with Art Deco-style geometric pattern, c. 1925-30. *Courtesy of Suzanjoy M. Checksfield.*

Hot pink "corduroy velour" negligee—surplice tie closing, trimmed with ostrich feathers and rows of hot pink fringe, c. 1925-30.

Blue silk jacquard kimono—polychromatic silk embroidery, embroidered pink satin cuffs. *Courtesy of Catherine Tobin. Photo by Bradley Schaeffer.*

NEGLIGEES

Also known as "hostess coats," elegant negligees were made of delicate fabrics such as corduroy velvet, crepe de chine, brocade, satin, georgette, rayon crepe, and serpentine crepe. Designed more for show than practicality, they were often made with long draped sleeves or trimmed with ruffles, rushing, silk fringe, lace, fur, ostrich feathers, eiderdown, *marabou,* or ribbon flowers.

COMBING SACQUE

Considered a luxury item, combing sacques (also known as dressing sacques) were loose waist-length jackets worn while styling the hair or applying makeup. They were made of satin or crepe de chine and decorated with lace.

KIMONOS

A passion for Oriental style, inspired a decade earlier by the *Ballet Russe* and fashion designer Paul Poiret, continued into the 1920s. This interest was reflected in the popularity of Japanese silk kimonos. They were elaborately decorated with beautiful hand embroidery in floral, bamboo, and bird motifs. Many women preferred wearing a kimono while playing the popular Chinese game called *mah-jongg,* which swept the nation during the 1920s.

26

BOUDOIR CAPS AND BANDEAUX

Delicate boudoir caps and *bandeaux* were worn to cover "rumpled or undressed hair" in the morning. They were usually made of pastel satin and trimmed with net ruffles, lace, or ribbon flowers. Human hair hairnets were worn to retain the marcel waves overnight.

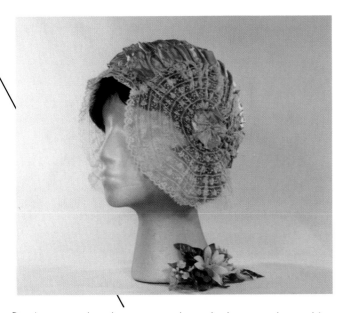

Boudoir cap—shirred mauve satin, lace wheels over each ear, ribbon flower in center. *Courtesy of Dorothy Byrnes.*

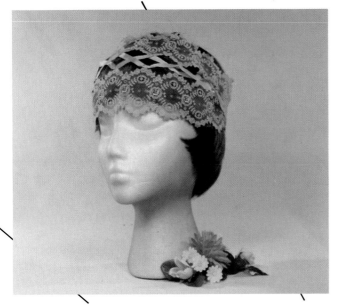

Boudoir *bandeau*—strips of ecru lace fastened together with latticework of peach satin ribbon.

SLIPPERS

Everyday house slippers were made of colorful felt. They were edged with top stitching, fur, or ribbon lacing and decorated with silk pompons or rosettes. Some styles had collars of contrasting quilted satin or checkered velvet.

Fancy mules or boudoir slippers were made of satin or brocaded fabric and trimmed with ostrich feathers, eiderdown, *marabou*, fur, and silk ribbon flowers.

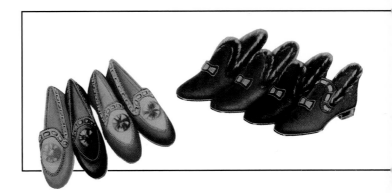

Felt bedroom slippers trimmed with pompons and fur. Charles William Stores, 1927-28.

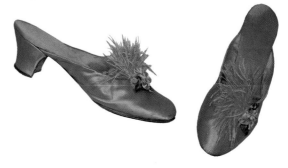

Hot pink satin mules—with ostrich feathers and pink silk ribbon flowers.

DESIGNERS OF LINGERIE

The Callot Soeurs designed ultra feminine nightgowns and chemises of gossamer silks, embellished with ribbon flowers and gold lace. Jeanne Lanvin, Mme. Jenny, and Martial et Armand also produced elegant lingerie during this period.

CHAPTER 3:
DAY WEAR

Because fashion is always evolving, the clothing worn in 1920 was remarkably different from that of 1929. Fashions of the first half of the decade were long, loose, and matronly, more suited to the mature figure. In stark contrast, the fashions of the second half of the decade were short, slender, and youthful, ideally suited to the new, flat-chested *garçonne* figure.

Four of the most popular colors of the decade were "Nile green" (medium green), "sunset orange" (light orange), "French blue" (medium blue) also known as "Copenhagen blue" or "gracklehead blue," and "maize" (light yellow). These were all soft muted shades which worked well together.

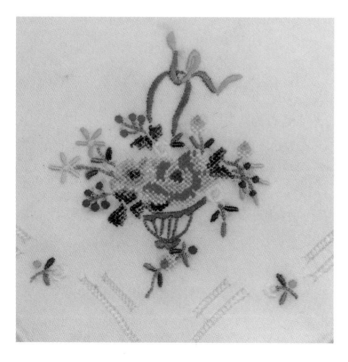

Handkerchief embroidered with rows of hemstitching and typical 1920s flower basket.

DRESSES

FORMAL AFTERNOON FROCKS

Formal afternoon dresses were worn to luncheons, teas, matinees, and tea dances. During the early twenties, day dresses often rivaled evening gowns with their luxurious fabrics and elaborate ornamentation.

Embroidery, whether rendered in silk floss or tiny beads, was the most popular form of ornamentation for dresses through out the decade. A few of the most common motifs were flower garlands, wreaths, flower baskets, bowknots, sunbursts, and abstract waterfalls. Geometric abstract designs also became popular after the introduction of Art Deco in 1925.

Machine embroidered trims, borders, and appliqués were also applied to dresses. During the teens and early twenties, narrow braid was stitched to garments in floral, scroll, and "vermicelli" (squiggly spaghetti) designs.

Printed fabrics were popular throughout the decade. Floral and geometric mini prints were the most popular. White or pastel backgrounds were used in summer, while darker colors were used in winter.

Ribbon was a popular form of ornamentation which found its way into every facet of a woman's wardrobe. Magazines such as *Ribbon Art* were published to illustrate the inexhaustible uses of the simple but feminine ribbon for the home seamstress.

In the late teens, the waistline was located just under the bust. It started its rapid decent in 1920, resting temporarily between the bust and the natural waist. It reached the natural waist in 1921, then quickly slipped to the hips in 1922, where it remained for the balance of the decade.

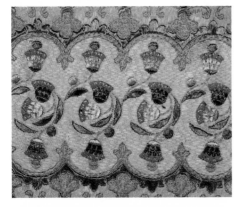

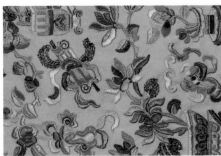

Machine embroidered trims with Chinese and Egyptian influence. *Courtesy of Suzanjoy M. Checksfield.*

Hemlines, in 1920, were just below the calf and remained there through 1922. In 1923 and 1924, they temporarily dropped to the ankle. Hems rose again in 1925, this time to the knee, creating what, at that time, was the shortest skirt in history! "Picot edging" was often used to bind the bottom edge of sheer dresses as it was softer and more supple than the conventional hem. It can be recognized by the tiny tufts along the edge of the fabric (about twelve per inch). They resemble the small picots or loops along the edges of picot ribbon, tatting, and other laces.

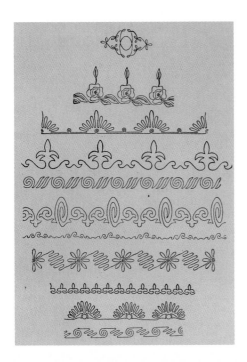

Dresses of the late teens and early twenties had roomy bodices without darts, which produced a saggy shapeless often blouson-effect. The most common necklines were the square, the boat, and the V-neck. Deep U, V, and square necklines were filled in with plastrons of the same or contrasting fabric. The popular horseshoe and tuxedo collars created strong vertical lines over the bust and formed a rectangular centerpiece which often received some form of decorative treatment. Shawl and sailor collars were also favored at this time. The most common sleeves were the fitted, the bell, and the cap sleeve.

Barrel-shaped underskirts ended below the calf, while shorter knee-length overskirts created a tunic-effect above (a carry-over from the teens). The one-piece "coat dress" was designed to look like a partially opened knee-length jacket worn over a dress. The jacket portion featured a tuxedo collar or was collarless.

Another popular skirt style was made in two sections—front and back. The sides of each section were allowed to drop three or four inches, creating points which hung below the rest of the hem. Other skirts had panels on each side which either hung even with or below the skirt hem.

Wide cummerbunds were often used, as well as fancy belts and sashes which incorporated ribbon cockades, pinwheels, flowers, *macramé*, beads, and tassels.

The bouffant *"robe de style,"* introduced by French fashion designer Jeanne Lanvin (circa 1915), offered an alternative to the tubular styles of the 1920s. (For further description of the robe de style see Chapter 4.)

Common fabrics for afternoon dresses were organdy, batiste, voile, georgette (silk crepe), satin, charmeuse, taffeta, and lace. They were often decorated with silk embroidery, beading, braid, lace, or *ruching.*

Typical designs for braided trim used on wearing apparel during the teens and early 20s. *Needle Art,* 1920.

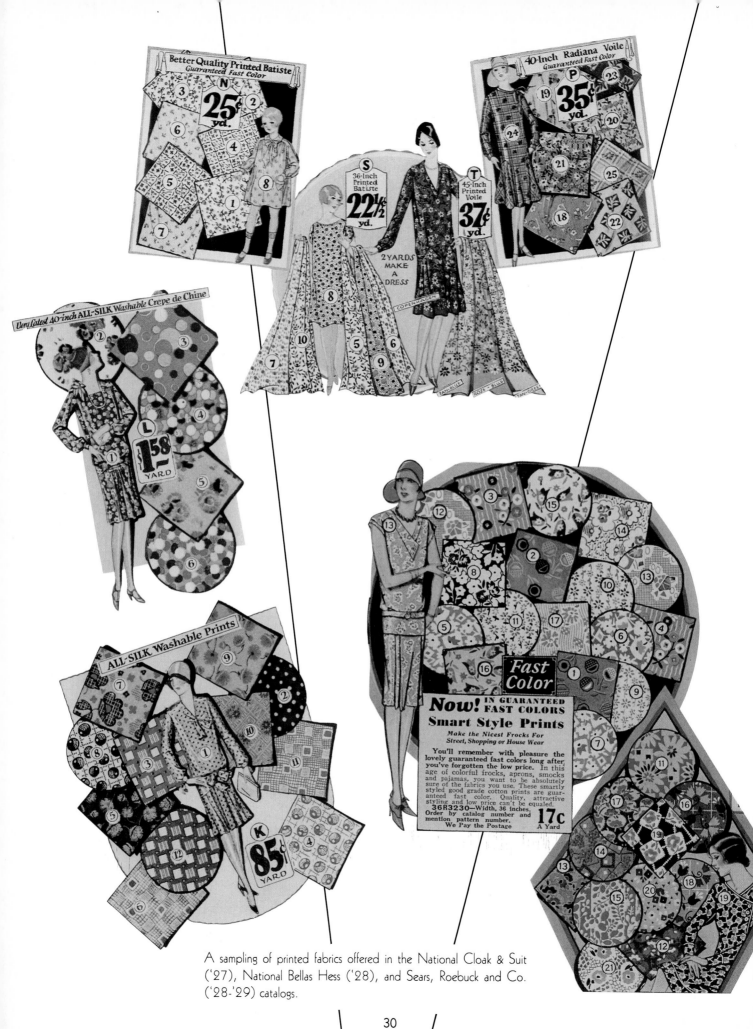

A sampling of printed fabrics offered in the National Cloak & Suit ('27), National Bellas Hess ('28), and Sears, Roebuck and Co. ('28-'29) catalogs.

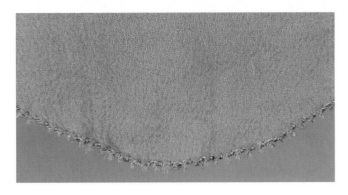

Picot edging at hem of orchid silk chiffon dress.

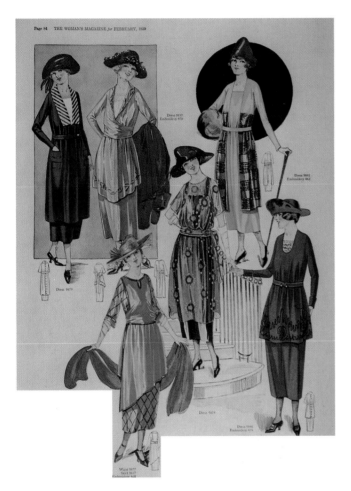

Five dresses feature tunics with shapeless bodices over barrel-shaped underskirts. Note: one yellow coat-dress. *The Woman's Magazine,* 2/20.

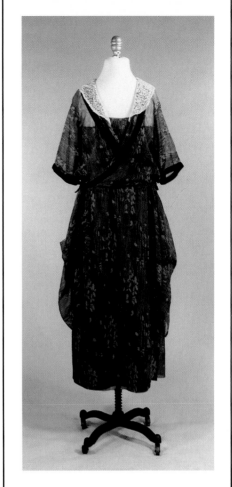

Afternoon dress of blue and pink patterned georgette, embroidered lace collar, velvet trim, late teens-early 20s. Label: Franklin Simon & Co.

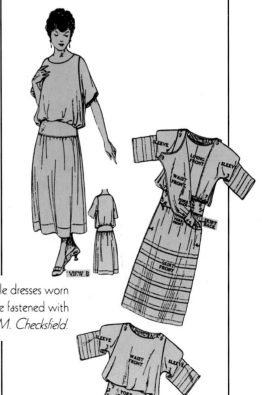

McCall pattern—illustrates construction of blouson-style dresses worn during the late teens and early 20s. (These dresses were fastened with multiple snaps and hooks) 1921. *Courtesy of Suzanjoy M. Checksfield.*

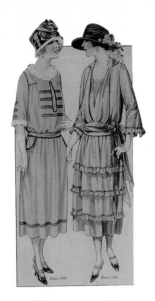
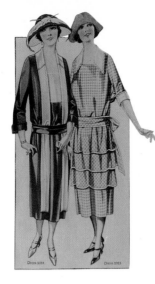

Afternoon dresses with loose bodices and gathered skirts. / Third— coat-dress with tuxedo collar. *Pictorial Review*, 5/22.

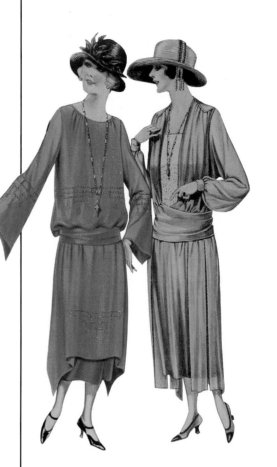

Day dresses. / Blouson bodice, bell sleeve, cummerbund, pointed hem. / Bishop sleeve, crisscross cummerbund, paneled skirt. *Pictorial Review*, 1922.

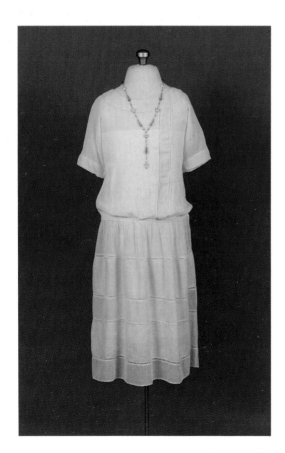

Day dress of white cotton voile trimmed with pink linen. *Courtesy of Cedar Crest Alumnae Museum, gift of Ellie Laubner. Photo by Bradley Schaeffer.*

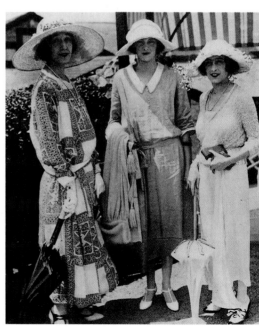

Ladies at Newport. Note: the wide-brimmed hats and long parasols. *Town & Country*, 8/22. *Courtesy of Judy Carpenter.*

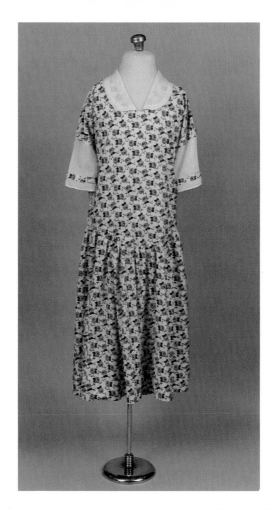

Floral print cotton day dress with gathered skirt. *Courtesy of Kemerer Museum, gift of Veleda Jones. Photo by Bradley Schaeffer.*

Ecru lace *robe de style* dress over Nile green silk slip, skirt held out at sides by built-in wire thigh hoops, decorated with silk ribbon flowers.

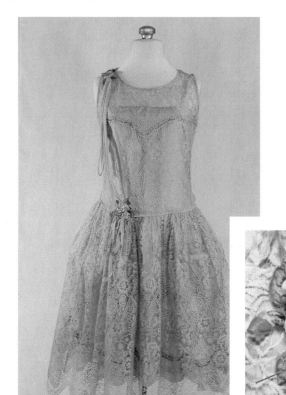

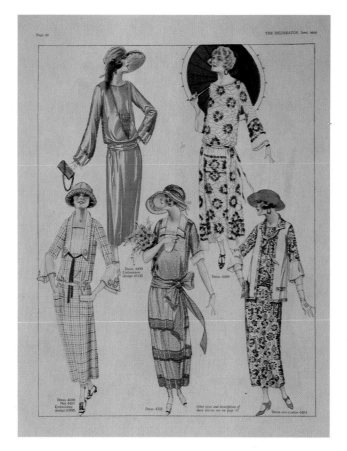

1923 and 1924

Dresses during this period were ankle-length tubes with dropped waists. The necklines, collars, and sleeves of the preceding years remained in favor.

The Russian-born painter/designer Sonia Delaunay created fashions from printed textiles which she created herself. Her bold Cubistic designs featured abstract shapes and patterns rendered in vivid hues, often on a white background.

Straight-line ankle-length dresses. Note: three deep filled-in necklines, two horseshoe collars, and bell sleeves (top right). *Delineator, 6/23.*

1925 and 1926

It was in 1925 that ladies' fashions crossed the threshold from "old fashioned" to what is now consider "modern." Dresses became streamlined and slender, without the excess fabric of previous years. Waistlines remained at the hip, while hemlines rose to the knee.

The most common necklines were the boat, the scoop, and the V-neck, while the Peter Pan, the shawl, and the Chelsea were popular collar styles. Common sleeves included the bishop, the fitted, and the cap sleeve. Many summer dresses, however, were sleeveless.

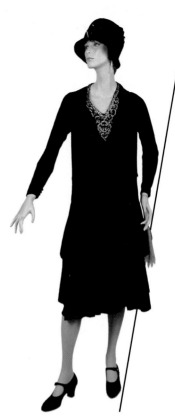

Black silk velvet afternoon dress with layered skirt, rhinestone trim at neckline. Label: Carolyn, New York, Paris. *Photo by Bradley Schaeffer.*

Blue satin dress with shirred flounce attached at an angle below hips, ecru lace trim. *Courtesy of Cedar Crest Alumnae Museum, gift of Ellie Laubner.*

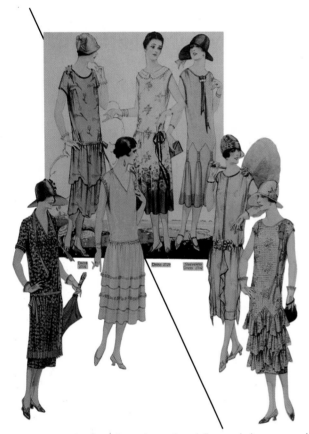

Summer afternoon frocks. Note: layered and flounced skirts, vertical ruffles, varied applications of ribbon. *Pictorial Review, 6/25.*

Orchid silk chiffon dress with matching satin slip, silk flocked flower, and scalloped picot hem edge. *Photo by Bradley Schaeffer.*

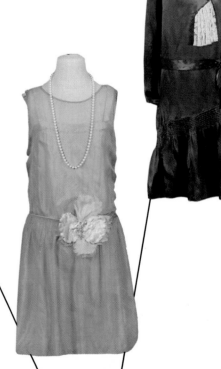

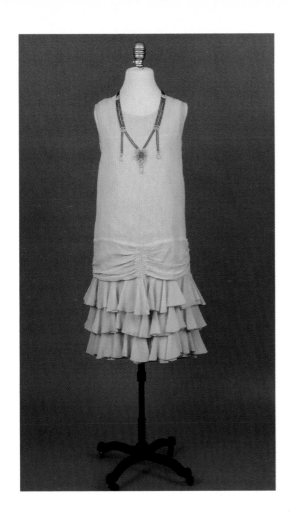

Yellow crepe dress with gypsy girdle and rows of flounces. *Courtesy of Kemerer Museum, gift of Suzanjoy M. Checksfield. Photo by Bradley Schaeffer.*

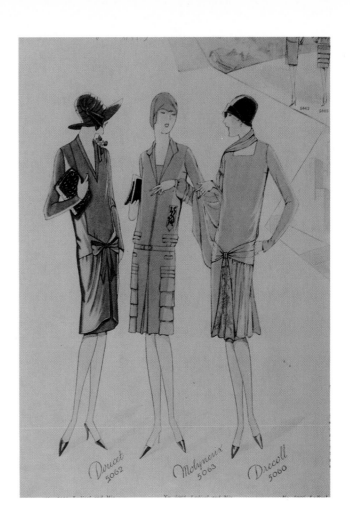

French designer frocks. / Doucet—bodice ties at hips. / Molyneux—rows of flounces. / Drécoll—gypsy girdle. *McCall's, 10/27.*

White georgette dress with gypsy girdle, bias-cut ruffles and flounces. c. 1927-29. *Courtesy of Rose Jamieson. Photo by Bradley Schaeffer.*

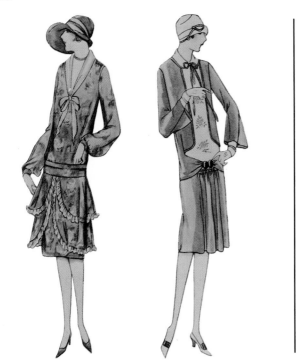

Afternoon dresses. / Shawl collar ending in bow, bishop sleeves, layered skirt. / Bell sleeves, bodice ends in mirror-image clasp. *McCall's, 6/26.*

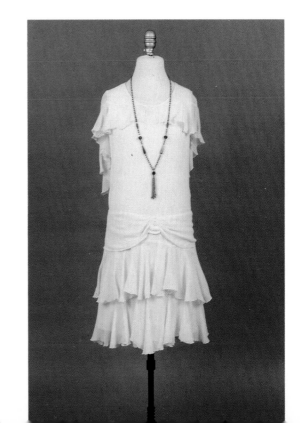

Skirts were often made from gathered layers or contained rows of gathered flounces. Others featured strips of fabric (two to three inches wide) which were attached to the skirt in vertical rows. Only one side of each strip was stitched to the skirt, allowing the other side to fall in undulating folds to a point at the hem. Bands of fur were another form of ornamentation applied to the hems of winter dresses.

The dropped waist was accented by narrow belts, or sashes which were tied in a bow over the right hip. In 1926, the "gypsy girdle" was introduced. It consisted of a wide sash fastened over the hips. It was gathered vertically at the center front, where it was often accented by a brooch or mirror-image clasp made of metal or bakelite. These clasps were often studded with rhinestones or marcasite. Another popular style featured a long bodice which was extended at the bottom to form two long streamers. The streamers were tied at the center of the dress at hip level.

Many of the fashion illustrations from 1924-1928 show long narrow ribbon bows placed at the shoulder, the hip, or the base of a collar. Some narrow shawl collars were extended at the bottom to form long streamers, which were tied in a bow. Silk chiffon or velvet flowers were often placed at the shoulder or the hip.

1927-1929

French *couturiere* Madeleine Vionnet created dresses using the "bias cut" (fabric cut on the diagonal). This set the trend for bias-cut skirts, flounces, jabots, cape collars, and cape sleeves, which fell in graceful fluted folds. This technique was used extensively during the 1930s. The bias cut required soft supple fabrics such as chiffon velvet, crepe de chine, silk satin, diaphanous chiffon, and lace. When cut on the bias these fabrics clung subtly to the body, which gave them shape. (For more on Madeleine Vionnet, see Chapter 4.)

Art Deco began to influence fashion as sweeping parallel and converging lines were added to dresses. These lines created the large geometric shapes that are so typical of Art Deco.

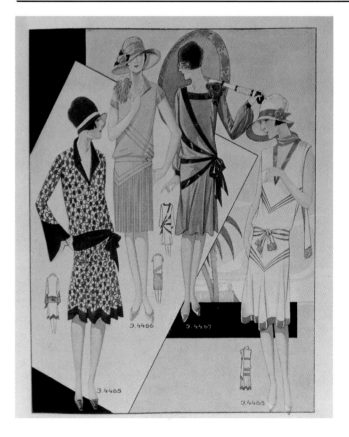

Art Deco-style dresses. Note: sweeping lines which divide dresses into geometric shapes, pleated and bias-cut skirts. *Reinach's Review of Fashion*, Paris, 1928. *Courtesy of Lehigh County Historical Society.*

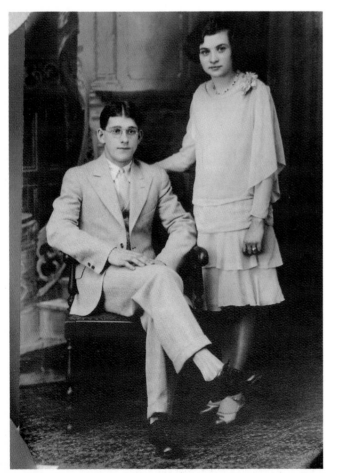

Young lady wears short beaded necklace, bias-cut drape over one sleeve, bias-cut flounced skirt, and two-toned shoes. Young man wears center part and round eyeglass frames.

Ensembles consisting of dresses or blouses and skirts with matching coats were popular during the second half of the decade. Many of the slender skirts had knife, box, or inverted pleats.

In late 1929, renowned French *couturier* Jean Patou returned the waist to its normal position. Dresses from 1929-1931 often have two waist seams, one at the normal waist and one at the hip. (Perhaps this was the fashion industry's way of creating a more gradual transition.) During the same year, Patou dropped the hemlines on day dresses to just below the calf. Longer skirts began to appear in fashion magazines of 1930, however, it took another year or so before mail-order houses like Sears, Roebuck caught up with this new length.

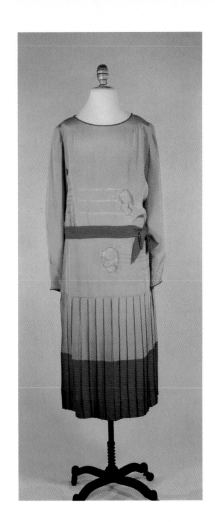

Tailored dress of rose and maroon silk crepe. Features knife-pleated skirt, horizontal hemstitching, lace inserts, c. 1929-30.

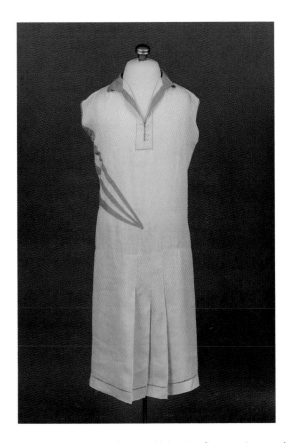

Pink linen dress with hemstitching and blue Art Deco-style trim. (Bears striking resemblance to previous illustration.) *Photo by Bradley Schaeffer.*

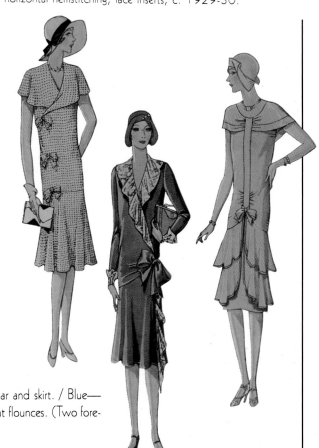

Afternoon frocks. / Yellow—bias-cut cape collar and skirt. / Blue—surplice style, bias-cut ruffles. / Orange—bias-cut flounces. (Two forehead hats.) *Pictorial Review,* 6/29.

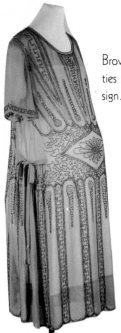

Brown georgette maternity dress decorated with brown beads. Note: ties at side for expansion. (Photographed on white for clarity of design.) *Courtesy of Cedar Crest Alumnae Museum, gift of Ellie Laubner.*

New calf-length bias-cut lace dress with dropped waist, ruffles at V-neck and sleeve. c. 1930-31. *Courtesy of Irene Cramer. Photo by Bradley Schaeffer.*

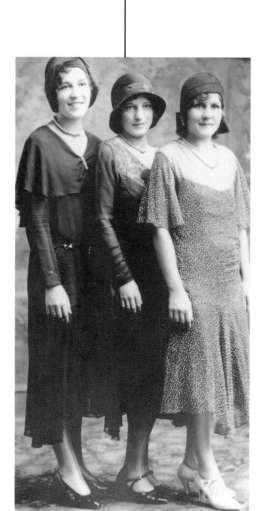

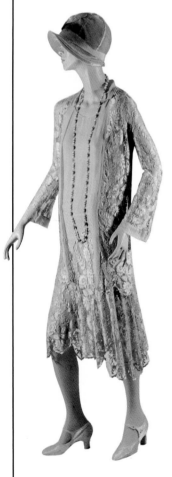

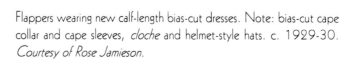

Flappers wearing new calf-length bias-cut dresses. Note: bias-cut cape collar and cape sleeves, *cloche* and helmet-style hats. c. 1929-30. *Courtesy of Rose Jamieson.*

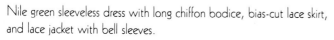

Nile green sleeveless dress with long chiffon bodice, bias-cut lace skirt, and lace jacket with bell sleeves.

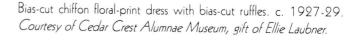

Bias-cut chiffon floral-print dress with bias-cut ruffles. c. 1927-29. *Courtesy of Cedar Crest Alumnae Museum, gift of Ellie Laubner.*

MORNING OR HOUSEDRESSES

Cotton housedresses were worn in the morning while carrying out household duties. Broadcloth, chambray, Indian head cloth, striped percale, and gingham checks and plaids were the most common fabrics used for housedresses. Piping, rickrack, and contrasting bindings were popular forms of trim.

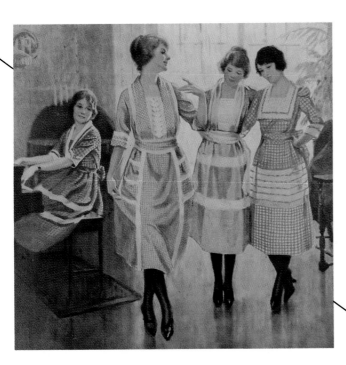

Ad for gingham-checked morning dresses by L'Aiglon. This illustration was evidently created before women abandoned black hose. *The Ladies' Home Journal*, 1/22.

1920-1924

While the sailor, Chelsea, shawl, tuxedo, and notched collars were the most common, collarless necklines were also offered. Housedresses had roomy gathered skirts with large utility patch pockets.

1925-1930

Housedresses, like other dresses, became shorter and more streamlined. Notched, pointed, and Chelsea collars were still in favor. Reversible-front "Hoover apron dresses" were made in the wraparound style, and featured a shawl collar. After one side was soiled, one could have a clean front surface again by simply reversing the sides. (Left over right, then became right over left.)

MATERNITY DRESSES

Pregnancy was no longer a time for seclusion. Maternity dresses, which followed the prevailing styles, were available from department stores and mail-order houses. They were made with numerous expandable pleats, or adjustable ties at the sides "to conceal the changes in figure."

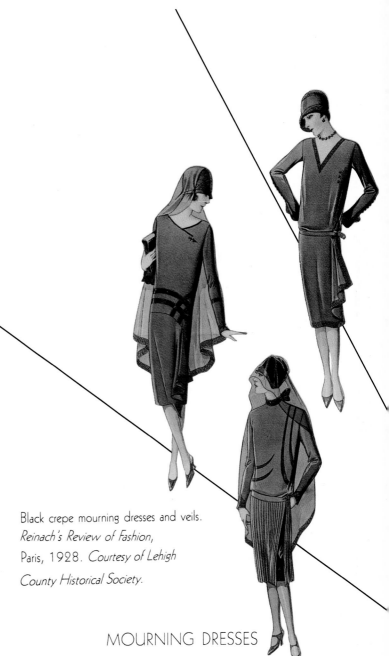

Black crepe mourning dresses and veils. *Reinach's Review of Fashion*, Paris, 1928. *Courtesy of Lehigh County Historical Society.*

MOURNING DRESSES

Although there had been a general loosening of mourning regulations since the Victorian era, black was still the accepted color for mourning clothing. A black wool or crepe dress was worn with black accessories. Women of the immediate family often wore black crepe or chiffon mourning veils pinned to their hats.

SUITS

1920-1922

Suits of wool worsted or serge featured shapeless thigh-length jackets with crisscross belts, and slender calf-length skirts. Detailing in the form of decorative buttons, top stitching, and embroidery was very common.

The popular convertible collar could be transformed from a broad cape-effect (when opened), to a high-standing choker collar which completely encircled the throat (when buttoned). These collars were often trimmed with fur. The Chelsea and notched collar styles were also common.

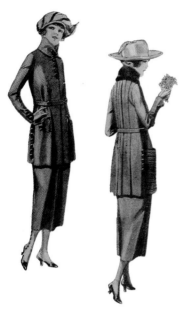

Suits with high-standing collars, loose tunic-style jackets with self belts, and slender skirts. Montgomery Ward, 1920-21.

1923-1924

Straight-line hip-length suit jackets created a dropped-waist effect, and covered the hip-length overblouses. Collar styles remained the same. Long straight skirts reached to the ankles.

"Coco" Chanel is best known for her "classic suit" which featured a long boxy collarless jacket and matching straight-line skirt. The edges of the jacket were trimmed with contrasting braid. The quilted lining of the jacket was made of the same coordinating silk as the matching blouse. Many of Chanel's jackets contain a signature chain which was placed

inside of the hem for weight. These suits were worn with her "illusion jewelry" consisting of gold chains, *faux* pearls, and large imitation gem stones.

1925-1930

Single and double-breasted straight-line jackets were paired with straight knee-length skirts. Some "edge-to-edge" jackets just met at the center front where they were held together by a link-button (resembling a cuff link). Suits became more slender and masculine with notched collars and peaked lapels. Many suits were pictured with men's four-in-hand neckties.

Typical colors for suits were navy, tan, brown, and black with white pin stripes. During the second half of the decade, suits were often worn with fur pieces draped over the shoulders. Irish-English born *couturier*, Edward Molyneux, designed soft tailored suits (navy in particular) which were ideal for work or for travel. His suits of printed silk or crepe featured thigh-length belted jackets with pleated skirts. His wearable styles and expert tailoring made him a favorite among his distinguished clientele.

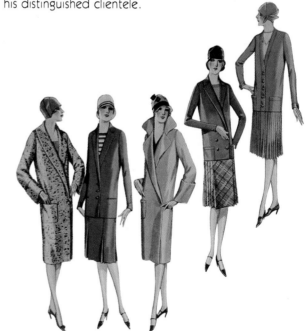

Single and double-breasted suits and surplice-style coats. *McCall Quarterly*, 1927.

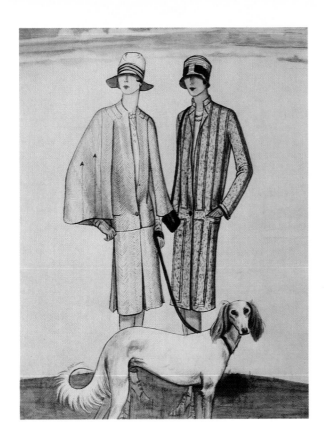

Styles by Chanel. / Variation of her classic collarless suit, herringbone, arrowhead stitching, worn with Reboux-style "gigolo" hat. / Tweed straight-line coat. *Vogue*, 4/27.

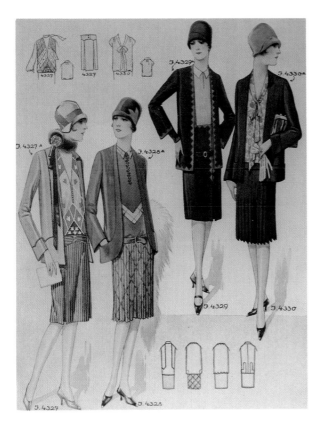

Chanel-style collarless suits—boxy jackets, pleated skirts. *Reinach's Review of Fashions*, Paris, 1928. *Courtesy of Lehigh County Historical Society.*

NEW TECHNOLOGY

The "automatic slide fastener" (later known as the zipper), began to appear on girl's leggings, boots, and luggage circa 1927 and 1928. Elsa Schiaparelli, an innovative designer always eager to try new technology, featured zippers in her 1933 line of fashions. By 1934 manufacturers were beginning to use zippers for women's jackets, and men's trousers and bathing suits.

When I first began collecting vintage clothing, I called my mother-in-law to ask when zippers were first used in clothing. (I figured this would be an invaluable aid when dating clothing.) She told me that, in 1934, she and my father-in-law took my husband's brother Bill (who was only three years old at the time) to a family wedding. He proceeded to demonstrate the new zipper in his Dad's fly to all of the guests at the wedding. This amusing incident remained indelibly printed on her mind for over 45 years.

In 1928, the Sanforized Company developed a process for pre-shrinking textiles before they were made into garments. This process was called sanforizing. I am reminded of another anecdote told to me by my mother-in-law describing life before sanforizing. She explained that one day on her way to work, she was caught in a downpour without an umbrella. When she arrived at work totally drenched, she looked down to discover that her dress had shrunk up above her knees. This length was totally improper for the work place, so she spent the rest of the day ducking behind office furniture and dodging her boss.

CHAPTER 4:
EVENING WEAR

The 1920s were a time of prosperity and conspicuous consumption. The extravagant gowns designed for lavish parties, dances, and night clubs were a reflection of this opulent era. They were made of such luxurious fabrics as silver and gold lamé, silk or metallic lace, chiffon velvet, crepe de chine, silk satin, georgette, and charmeuse. Solid-colors were usually preferred over patterned fabrics, with the accent provided by gold and silver embroidery, sparkling *rocaille*, glittering *paillettes*, and dazzling *diamanté*.

Beads were often applied to sheer gowns made of net, chiffon, or georgette. They were then worn over an opaque slip of the same or a contrasting color. While most beading was done by machine, labor-intensive hand beading was painstakingly produced by the famous *couture* houses. Home seamstresses also beaded garments using patterns provided by needlework magazines of the period.

In 1920, the waistline was placed slightly above its natural position. It then fell to the hips in 1922, where it remained until the end of the decade.

The hemline for evening gowns followed the lead of daytime dresses. It rested just below the calf from 1920 through 1922. In 1923 and 1924, it dropped temporarily to the ankle, only to rise again to the knee in 1925, where it remained for the balance of the decade. Irregular hems of all kinds were popular throughout the 1920s. They were created through attached panels, handkerchief squares, asymmetrical draping, zigzag and scalloped cuts, and diamond-shaped godets.

1920-1922

The loose blouson-style bodice featured either a shallow boat neckline, or a deep U or V-neckline filled in with a contrasting plastron. The waistline was usually trimmed with a wide cummerbund or sash.

An irregular hem was created by allowing the material at the side of skirt to fall into points below the hemline. The romantic handkerchief hem, introduced in the early teens, was a popular favorite with teenage girls during the first half of the decade. It was made of large filmy squares of fabric resembling handkerchiefs. Each square was fastened by one of the corners to the waistband of the dress, creating numerous soft points at the hem. This technique was frequently used by designer Madeleine Vionnet.

The Callot Soeurs (Callot sisters) were partners in one of Paris's leading couture houses from 1916 to 1937. They were daughters of a lace maker and an antique dealer specializing in old fabric and lace. It is not surprising then, that the sisters embellished their sheer ultra feminine designs with one-of-a-kind Rococo-style embroidery and antique lace. They were also the first to use gold and silver lamé.

Another eminent designer was Mariano Fortuny, a Spaniard who lived in Venice. He was an accomplished painter, inventor, chemist, and fashion designer whose garments did not follow the trends of mainstream *haute couture*, nor did he advertise in fashion magazines of the period. His timeless garments were nevertheless admired and sought after by fashion-conscious women around the world.

In 1906, Fortuny created what he called the "Delphos" dress, a delicate floor-length gown, worn for afternoon or evening. He patterned this gown after the columnar Ionic *chitons* worn by the women of ancient Greece. It was made of lustrous silk which he dyed by hand, using natural vegetable dyes. The results were exquisite silks in soft subtle shades of pink, blue, green, gold, and rust. He then pleated the delicate fabric into tiny mushroom pleats, using an undisclosed process which he patented in 1909.

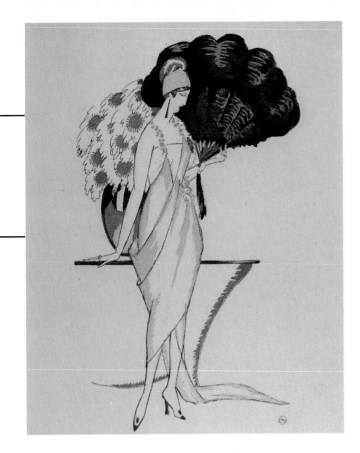

Evening gown with unusual spiral draping by Worth, 1920.

He created many one and two-piece variations of this gown over his forty-three year career (1906-1949). Common features included a drawstring neckline; laced shoulder seams; fagoted side seams; short, long, or batwing sleeves; and small Venetian glass beads which were fastened along the edges of the dresses and tunics for weight. Due to the elasticity of the pleats, these supple gowns acquired their shape from the uncorseted feminine figure. To retain their pleats, the gowns were twisted like a rope, then coiled into small round boxes (eight inches in diameter) for sale or for storage.

To accompany these attractive gowns, Fortuny designed velvet evening wraps, cloaks, capes, and jackets with wide graceful sleeves. He hand dyed the silk velvet which he later stenciled or block printed with gold or silver paint. The patterns and patina of these lovely garments were reminiscent of medieval and Renaissance tapestries.

All of Fortuny's garments have the understated elegance and classic design which makes his work as wearable today as it was four decades ago. His garments were regarded as status symbols during the 1920s and 1930s, and are now considered rare treasures, eagerly sought after by collectors around the world.

The romantic *robe de style* was introduced by French designer Jeanne Lanvin, circa 1915. It consisted of a basque bodice with a broad neckline, and an oval bouffant skirt. (The fullness at the sides of the skirt was supported by built-in wire thigh-hoops.) This nostalgic gown resembled the wide Spanish *infanta*-style dresses of the 17th century. For this reason, it was often worn with a Spanish shawl, a large decorative back comb, or a lace *mantilla*. The *robe de style* was also reminiscent of the 18th century *robe à la française,* which was supported at the sides by a wire undergarment called a *pannier*. Therefore, it was also referred to as a "*pannier* dress."

The *robe de style* was usually made of silk taffeta, organdy, velvet, satin, or metallic lace. Lanvin preferred to use solid colors (particularly a deep shade of robin's egg blue, which became known as "Lanvin blue"). These solid colors became the backdrop for a spectacular crescendo of silver embroidery and beadwork which was usually concentrated in one area of the gown. Her favorite motifs for this ornamentation were flowers, ribbon bows, sunbursts, and Art Deco shapes, which were executed in rhinestones, sequins, and beads. She also made use of silk flowers, colorful free-flowing ribbons, and taffeta appliqués which appeared to float over sheer layers of tulle. Shorter versions of the *robe de style* were especially popular for teenage girls. Surprisingly, this romantic style remained in favor until the late 1930s, providing a feminine alternative to the androgynous tubular styles of the 1920s. (For a *robe de style* wedding gown see Chapter 5.)

Lanvin is also remembered for her popular fragrances, "My Sin" (1925) and "Arpège" (1927). She opened branch boutiques in the French resort towns of Nice, Cannes, and Biarritz where she carried a range of children's wear, lingerie, and men's accessories (introduced in 1926).

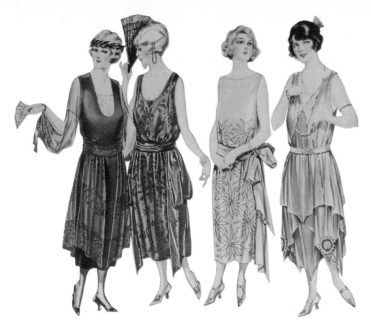

Evening gowns with loose bodices, sashes, irregular and handkerchief hems. Note: laurel and beaded headbands, back comb. *Pictorial Review*, 12/21.

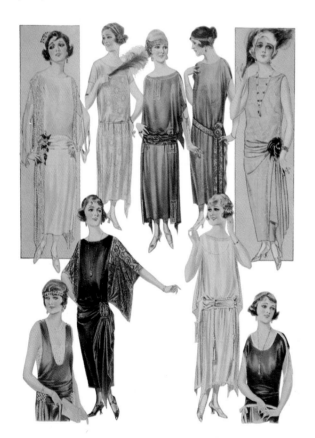

Loose-fitting evening gowns with boat necklines, decorative sashes, draping, and uneven hems. Note: headbands, back comb, and long necklaces. *Pictorial Review*, 7/22.

Green georgette dress decorated with silver-lined bugle and seed beads, four beaded panels over the skirt. Note: resemblance to previous illustrations. *Courtesy of F. Paul Laubner.*

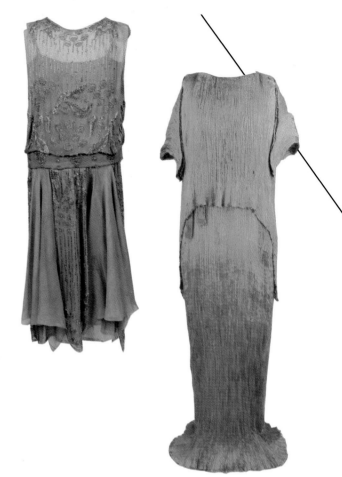

Rust pleated silk *Delphos* dress with lacing over shoulders, Venetian glass beads along hem of tunic. Fortuny name stenciled on sash. *Courtesy of Mary Anne Faust (Yesterday's Delights).*

1923 and 1924

Gowns became slender ankle-length tubes, often featuring the popular boat neckline. Gowns with deep U or V-shaped necklines were worn over colorful straight-cut slips. The waistline dropped to the hip where it was accented by a decorative sash or was left undefined. Asymmetrical effects were produced by draping the excess fabric to one hip, where it was embellished with a rhinestone ornament, a large bow, or a *chou*.

The French designer, Jean Patou, frequently trimmed the edges of his fashions with a thick band of luxurious fur. This dramatic effect was often copied by other designers who attached bands of fox, seal, chinchilla, kolinsky, mink-dyed muskrat, monkey, and even skunk to the hemlines of their gowns.

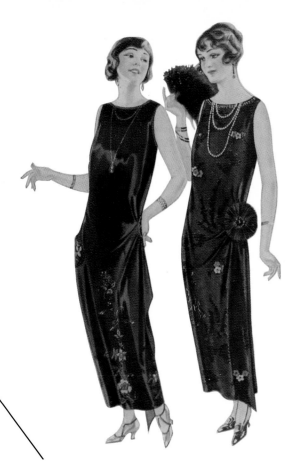

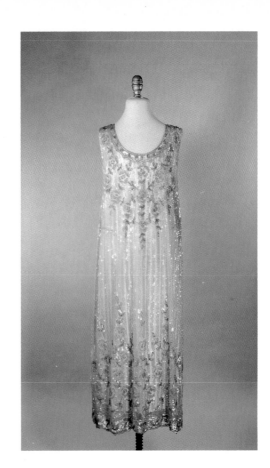

Ankle-length draped silk velvet evening gowns with boat necklines and silk floral embroidery. *Pictorial Review*, 11/23.

French designer gown of silk chiffon, crazy quilt pattern, embroidered with gold metallic thread, bodice decorated with seed beads, draped fabric falls below hem. Signed: Revellin, 83295. *Courtesy of F. Paul Laubner.*

Beige net gown covered with cream iridescent sequins and beaded green and terra cotta floral design, c. 1923-24. *Courtesy of F. Paul Laubner.* Photo by Bradley Schaeffer.

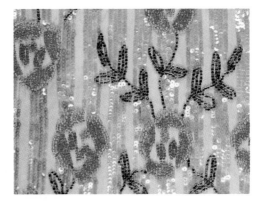

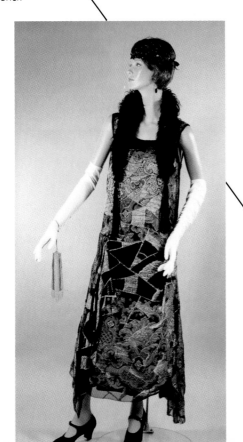

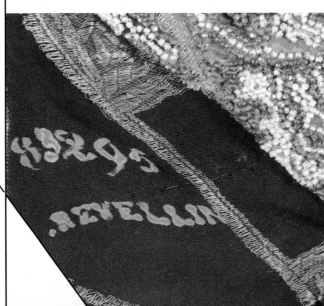

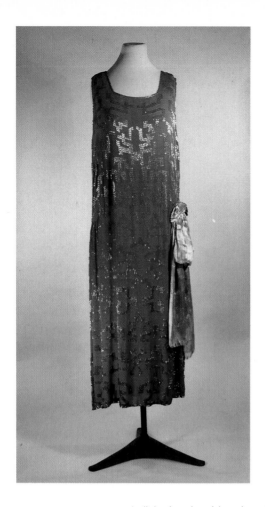

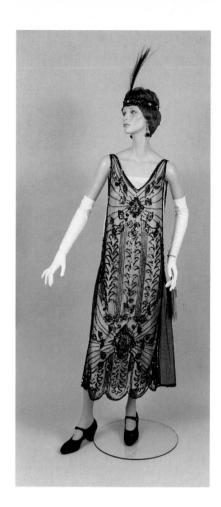

Cranberry crepe evening gown embellished with gold, red, and blue bugle beads and gold lamé sash. *Courtesy of the family of Helen Harleman Chase.*

Black net dress with blue iridescent sequins and bugle beads over turquoise slip. *Photo by Bradley Schaeffer.*

Gray silk crepe gown decorated with sequins, small silver balls, and beaded fringe. *Courtesy of Cedar Crest Alumnae Museum, on loan from Priscilla Gerlach Rosendale.*

Black georgette gown with rhinestones applied in diamond pattern, 1924. *Courtesy of Margaretha J. Laubner.*

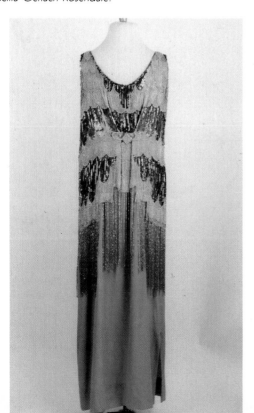

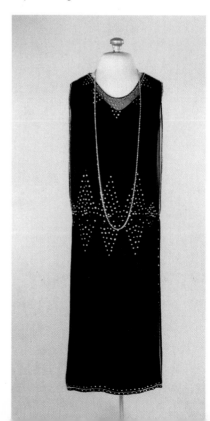

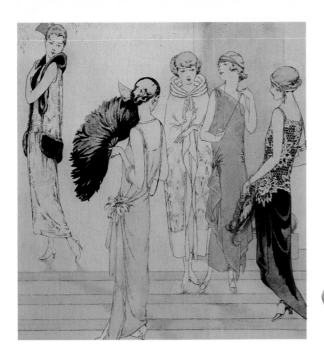

Long tubular gowns and white evening cape with ermine collar and silver embroidery. Note: trains, fur trim, side draping, combs, and *bandeaux. Ladies' Home Journal,* 11(late)/22.

Ankle-length evening gowns including a *robe de style.* Note: the *bandeaux* and beaded sunburst motif. *Elite Style,* 4/23.

Red satin evening dress with asymmetrical draping, rhinestone ornament. *Courtesy of Kemerer Museum, gift of Veleda Jones.*

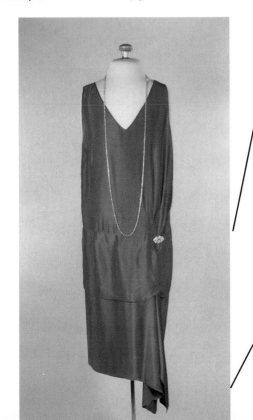

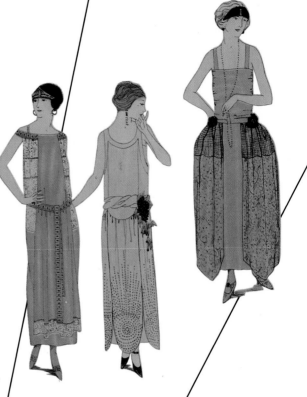

1925 and 1926

The hemlines on evening dresses rose to the knee in 1925, where they remained until the end of the decade.

The "gypsy girdle," a popular feature of 1920s dresses, consisted of a wide sash fastened over the hips. It was gathered vertically at the center front where it was often accented with a large rhinestone brooch or "mirror-image" clasp. It was also fashionable to add gathered panels to the sides of skirts.

The evening dresses most often associated with the 1920s are those containing rows of silk or beaded fringe. They were primarily produced during the years 1925 through 1928, and are quite collectible.

In 1926, skirts were cut from a full circle of soft sheer fabric, or they contained godet inserts which created a slight flare at the hem. Other skirts featured vertical strips of fabric (two to three inches wide) which were fastened to the skirt along one edge only. This allowed the opposite edge to fall in soft undulating folds to the hem.

Another popular style featured a long hip-length bodice which was extended to form two long ends. These ends were then tied in a bow or square knot at the center front.

In 1926, plunging V or U-shaped necklines were cut from the backs of evening gowns, a sophisticated style which continued into the 1930s.

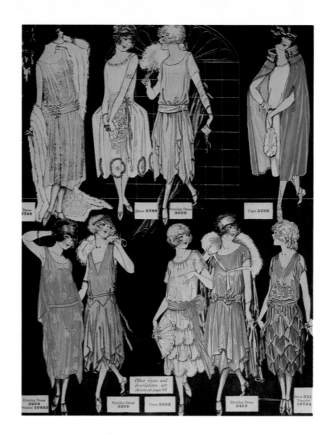

Flapper dresses featuring *robe de style* (top row, 2nd from left), evening cape, and handkerchief skirts. Note: four *bandeaux. Butterick Quarterly*, Fall 1922. *Courtesy of Phillis Hallett.*

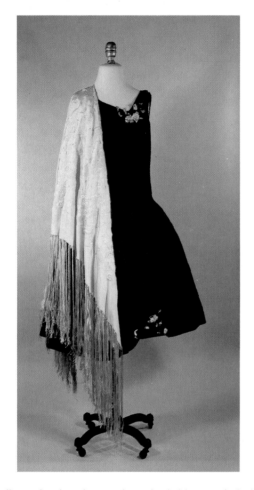

Black taffeta *robe de style* party dress, skirt held out with thigh hoops, asymmetrical neck and hemlines trimmed with pink ribbon flowers, 1926. *Courtesy of Margaretha J. Laubner.* / Peach embroidered silk shawl.

Scoop and V-neck evening gowns trimmed with panels, flounces, godets, and ties. *Pictorial Review,* 10/25.

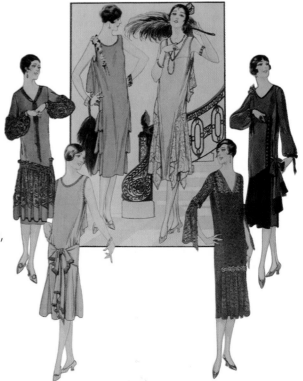

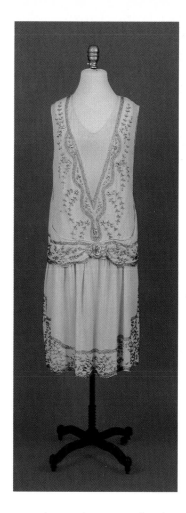

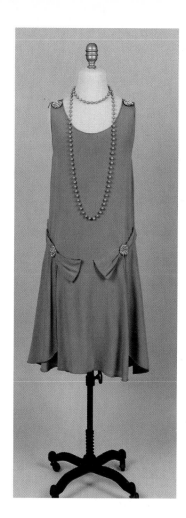

Yellow crepe evening dress with gypsy girdle, decorated with silver-lined seed beads, c. 1927-29. *Courtesy of Roseann Ettinger (Remember When...). Photo by Bradley Schaeffer.*

Turquoise crepe dress with four ornamental rhinestone buttons. *Courtesy of Kemerer Museum, gift of Mrs. Edmund Martin. Photo by Bradley Schaeffer.*

Black georgette evening gown over black slip, decorated with black, blue, and purple seed beads, 1925. *Courtesy of Pauline Weber.*

Black georgette evening dress, delicate floral design created with blue, pink, and peach seed beads. *Courtesy of Grace Voorhees Howells. Photo by Bradley Schaeffer.*

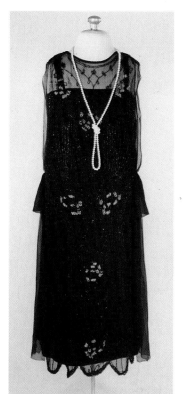

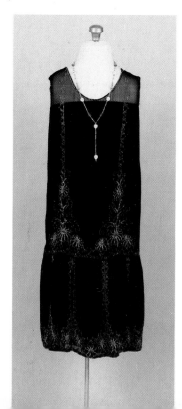

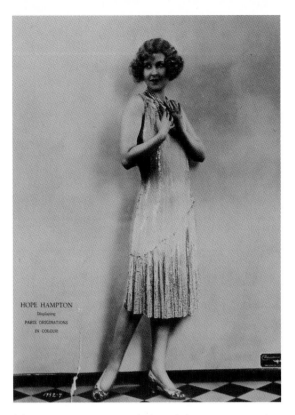

Hope Hampton wearing a wavy bob and glittering evening dress with beaded fringe.

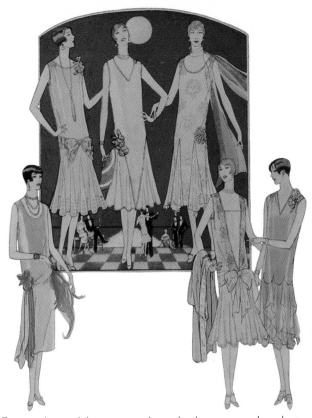

Evening dresses. Note: two with circular skirts, two with godet inserts, two with bows, and one with handkerchief panels. *Butterick Quarterly*, summer 1926. *Courtesy of Rose Jamieson.*

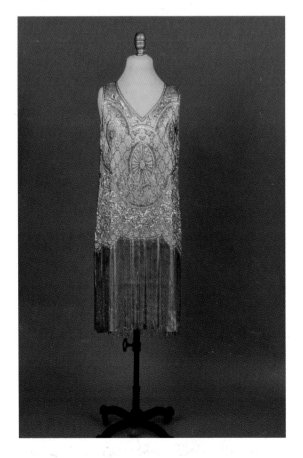

Light green satin evening dress decorated with silver sequins, bugle beads, rhinestones, and beaded fringe. *Courtesy of Warren Hills Regional High School, gift of Grace Chardavoyne. Photo by Bradley Schaeffer.*

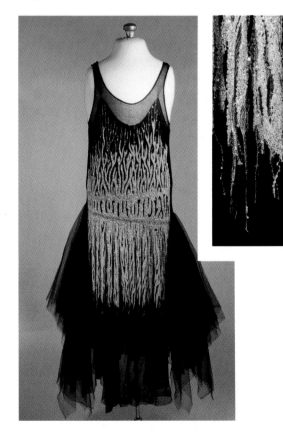

Black net designer gown decorated with elaborate pattern of tiny silver balls and seed beads, black net skirt. Purchased in Paris, 1926. *Courtesy of Richard Groman.*

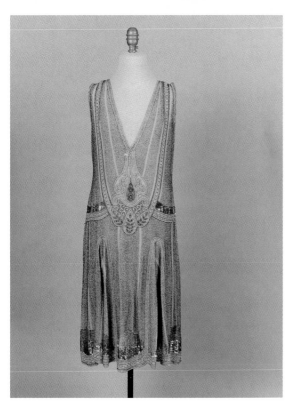

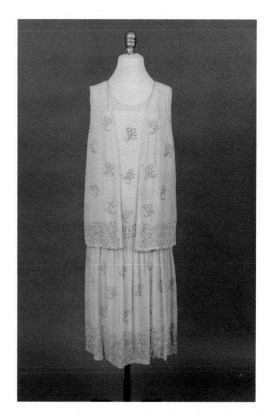

Gray crepe designer dress covered with rhinestones, pearls, embossed sequins, and silver-lined seed beads (all applied by hand), four godet inserts in skirt. *Photo by Bradley Schaeffer.*

Peach crepe evening dress with matching sleeveless jacket, decorated with clear rhinestones. Worn by perspective bride to engagement party. Label: Lord and Taylor, New York. *Photo by Bradley Schaeffer.*

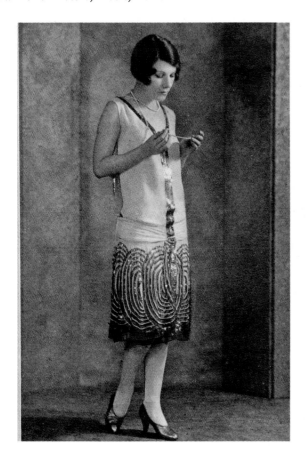

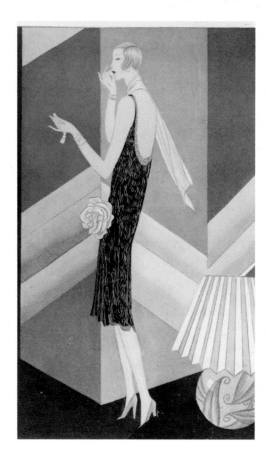

White chiffon evening dress with gold sequins, worn with long strand of pearls. *Town & Country, 9/26. Courtesy of Judy Carpenter.*

Black lace evening dress by Chanel featuring plunging neckline (in back), accented with chiffon scarf and silk flower. *Vogue, 5/1/26. Courtesy of Richard Groman.*

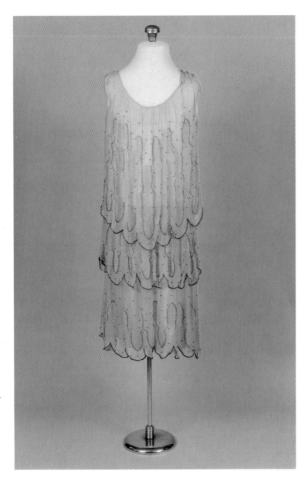

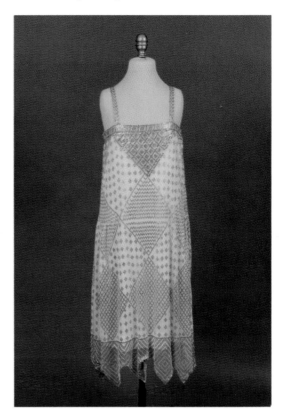

Evening dress of Egyptian Assuit cloth, Art Deco diamond pattern created with tiny pieces of metal. (For information on Assuit stoles, see chapter 7.) *Photo by Bradley Schaeffer.*

Yellow silk chiffon two-piece dress—loose scalloped bodice over a dress with two scalloped flounces, trimmed with round black beads and white frosted bugle beads. *Courtesy of F. Paul Laubner. Photo by Bradley Schaeffer.*

Black net evening gown with zigzag hem, decorated with gold seed beads and black sequins, photographed over pink slip.

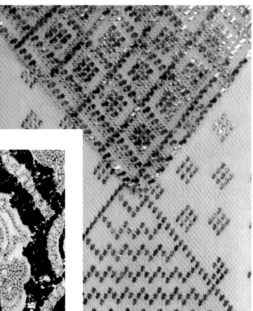

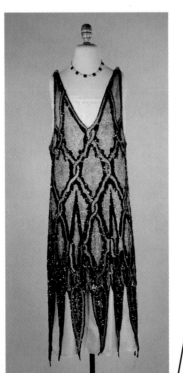

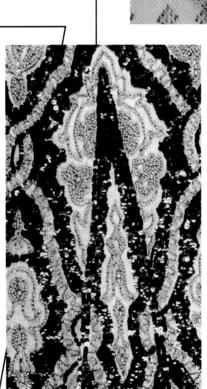

Many skirts of this period featured draped panels which fell into soft points at the hem. Multi-layered skirts were common, as well as skirts with scalloped or zigzag hems.

The gypsy girdle remained a popular feature, along with the wide sash which was tied in an enormous bow over one hip.

The bias cut was used extensively by the influential French designer Madeleine Vionnet. She set the trend for bias-cut bodices, skirts, flounces, jabots, cape collars, and cape sleeves which were prevalent from 1927 through the 1930s. This technique helped to soften the look and relieve the tedium of the severe rectangular silhouette. The bias cut required soft supple fabrics such as filmy chiffon, georgette, silk velvet, crepe de chine, and silk satin. Vionnet's garments clung subtly to the body, which gave them shape, then fell in graceful fluted folds to the hem.

Vionnet's talent lay principally in the unique cut of her garments, which she masterfully designed on a small articulated mannequin. This complex construction made her styles quite difficult to duplicate. Because of the natural elasticity which the bias cut provided, Vionnet's dresses could be pulled over the head with no need for fastenings. (See Chapter 5 for a Vionnet wedding gown.)

In late 1928, the unusual bi-level hemline, a favorite of the designer Louiseboulanger, fell just below the knee in front and below the calf in back.

This ephemeral style gave way, in late 1929, when Jean Patou lowered the entire hemline to the ankle for evening, and raised the waistline to its natural position. Ironically, the short economical styles of the twenties came to an end at a time when many people lost their fortunes overnight, due to the stock market crash.

Until 1929, American motion picture stars wore their own clothing on the silver screen. The sudden drop in hemlines dictated by Paris caught the American motion picture industry by surprise. It was left with brand new movies featuring short outdated dresses. To prevent this regrettable situation from reoccurring, movie moguls hired their own costume designers to provide them with up-to-the-minute sophisticated styles with which to dazzle their audiences.

Other French designers and couture houses of the 1920s included Jacques Doucet, Lucien Lelong, Mme. Premet, Drécoll, Jenny, Augustabernard, and Edward Molyneux. Elegant evening gowns were also the specialty of New York designer Eldridge Manning.

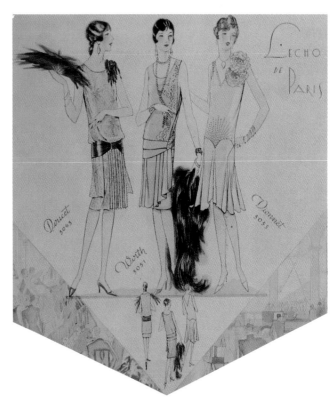

Three French designer dresses. / Doucet—gypsy girdle, pleats. / Worth—asymmetrical pleats. / Vionnet—beaded Deco sunburst design and bias-cut skirt. *McCall's*, 10/27.

Peach georgette evening dress with circular skirt, trimmed with silver-lined bugle beads, peach seed beads, and rhinestones. (Note striking resemblance to Vionnet dress in previous illustration.) *Courtesy of Roberta Wickley, (R&R Collectibles). Photo by Bradley Schaeffer.*

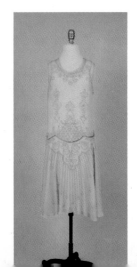

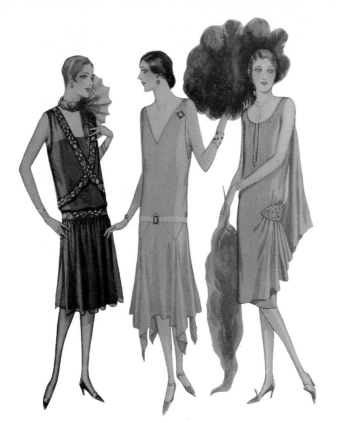

CARE OF BEADED DRESSES

If stored on a hanger, the weight of heavy beading can break the shoulder seams of fragile beaded dresses. Gravity also tugs at the beads, eventually weakening the beading threads. Therefore, it is recommended that beaded dresses be stored flat in acid free boxes, with acid free tissue paper, or wrapped in unbleached muslin. (Ordinary paper, cardboard, and wood contain acids which burn textiles with which they come into contact for any length of time.)

Plastic bags are not recommended for the storage of clothing as they trap moisture and promote the growth of mold and mildew. Plastic also tends to dull the color of sequins.

Many of the clear seed beads were lined with silver to enhance their sparkle. Over the years the silver tarnishes, thereby giving the beads a dark gray appearance.

Three French designer evening gowns. / Lanvin—peasant trim. / Vionnet—superb example of Vionnet's talents with the bias cut. / Worth—asymmetrical draping and rhinestone studded patch. *McCall Quarterly*, summer 1927.

Ultra-sophisticated gowns by French designer, Augusta-bernard. Note: plunging neckline (in back), jeweled belt, round bias-cut godets at sides which create uneven hem. *McCall's*, 4/29.

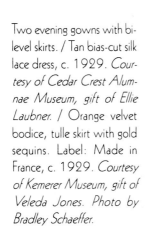

Two evening gowns with bi-level skirts. / Tan bias-cut silk lace dress, c. 1929. *Courtesy of Cedar Crest Alumnae Museum, gift of Ellie Laubner.* / Orange velvet bodice, tulle skirt with gold sequins. Label: Made in France, c. 1929. *Courtesy of Kemerer Museum, gift of Veleda Jones. Photo by Bradley Schaeffer.*

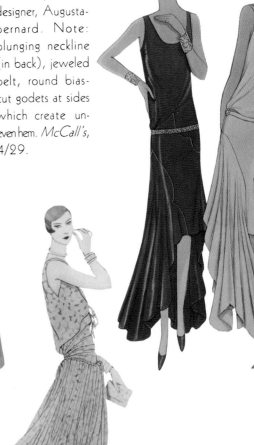

Red silk velvet evening dress with asymmetrical draping and rhinestone studded patches. (Note similarity to Worth dress in previous illustration.) c. 1927. *Courtesy of Theresa Schouten.*

Gown with bi-level skirt created by French designer Louiseboulanger. *Vogue*, 4/27. (This style became popular in late 1928-29.)

CHAPTER 5:
BRIDAL WEAR

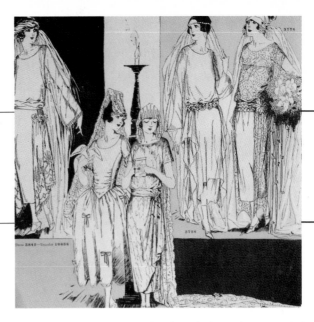

Bridal fashions with added panels, draped skirts, decorative sashes. Bottom left—*robe de style* worn with back comb and Spanish mantilla. Bottom right—Egyptian-style headpiece. *Butterick Quarterly,* 1922. *Courtesy of Phillis Hallett.*

WEDDING GOWNS

Wedding gowns were patterned after evening gowns of the period, featuring many of the same details and elements of design. Some brides preferred gowns made of plain white satin, georgette, chiffon, or crepe de chine; while others were influenced by the glitz and glitter of the period. Brides from well-to-do families often wore gowns of silver lamé decorated with metallic lace, silver embroidery, rhinestones, sequins, crystal beads, or pearls.

Wedding gowns commonly featured a dropped waist or they had no defined waist at all. The boat and the scooped necklines were the most popular. Long, short, or no sleeves were all considered acceptable. Trains, when they were added, were usually rectangular in shape.

1920-1922

Bridal gowns featured blouson-style bodices with skirts ending just below the calf. Decorative sashes were placed at, or slightly below, the natural waist. Short set-in, kimono, or bell sleeves were the most common.

Irregular hems were created using a variety of techniques. The handkerchief hem (introduced during the teens) continued to be a favorite. Long gathered panels were added to the sides of skirts, or the fabric of the skirt was draped to the right hip where it was embellished with a beaded ornament or silk flowers. Another technique involved open side seams which allowed the fabric to fall in graceful undulating folds, ending in points which dipped below the hemline.

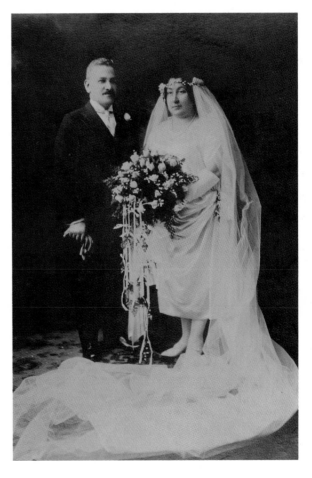

White satin gown with fabric draped to right hip, veil attached to wreath of wax blossoms, elbow-length gloves. c.1921-22.

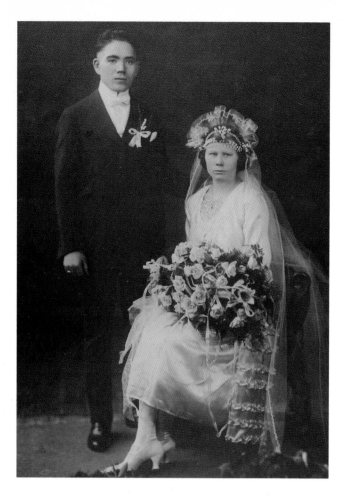

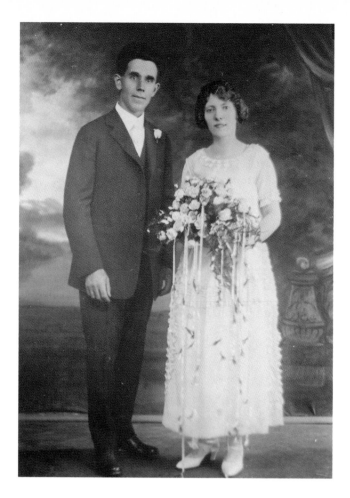

"Radiant" bride wearing fan-shaped headpiece, white satin gown with filled in neckline, horizontal rows of *ruching*, and pointed shoes with Louis heels. c. 1921-22.

Bride wears white gown with ruffled trim and white strap shoes, 7/29/23. *Courtesy of Emma and Eric Nordeen.*

1923-1924

Wedding gowns became long slender tubes, usually ending at the ankles. Dropped waists were accented by the use of decorative sashes. Draped skirts remained in vogue. Narrow rows of ruffles or ruching were often applied to the neckline, sleeves, and hem.

Attendant's gown flanked by two wedding gowns. / Satin embellished with silver and white embroidery and crystal beads. / Crepe trimmed with lace, looped mandarin bands. / Satin and chiffon with gold and silver embroidery and seed pearls. *Elite Style*, 5/23.

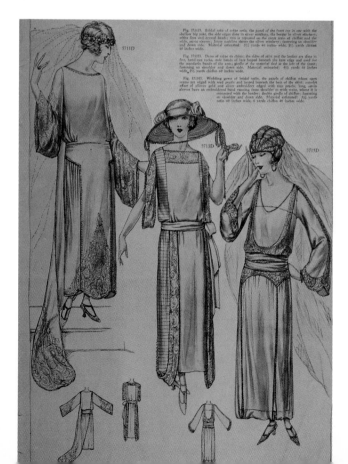

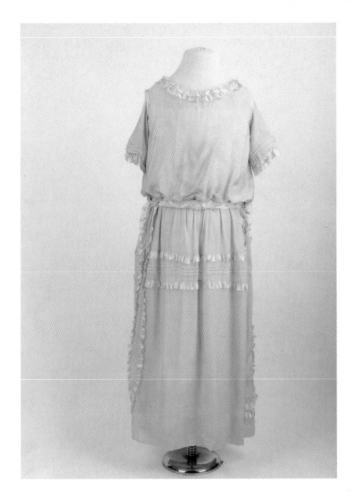

Blouson-style crepe de chine wedding gown with satin ruffles and braided waistband (from accompanying portrait) 7/29/23. *Courtesy of Emma and Eric Nordeen.*

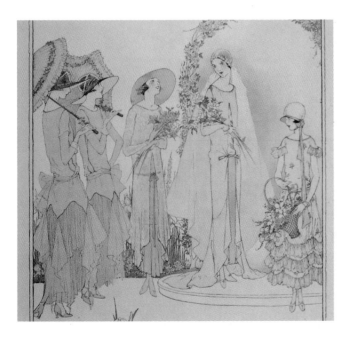

Two bridesmaids wear straw picture hats and carry flower decked parasols in lieu of flowers. / Bride wears veil gathered over head, long tubular gown. / Flower girl carries typical 20s flower basket. *The Ladies' Home Journal,* 4/24.

1925-1926

Dropped waists were accented with tied sashes, silk flowers, or gypsy girdles. Long bodices with extended streamers were tied in a bow, or fastened with a clasp at the center front.

Knee-length gowns were considered acceptable, however, many gowns were slightly longer. Soft supple fabrics were used for circular skirts, which fell in gentle fluted folds. Triangular or diamond-shaped godets were inserted into the hems of skirts, creating a slight flare. Vertical ruffles also added a soft feminine touch.

Jeanne Lanvin is noted for her fanciful *robe de style* wedding gowns, which were worn throughout the decade. The bouffant skirts created a romantic feminine air. (See Chapter 4 for more details on the *robe de style.*)

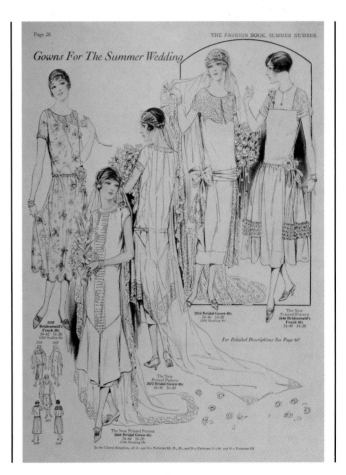

Three wedding dresses flanked by two attendants' dresses. Note: coronet headpiece in center, *robe de style* on the far right. *The Fashion Book,* Summer 1925.

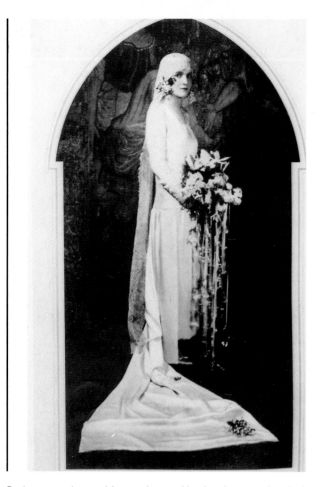

Bride wears a lace veil fastened around her head accented with clusters of flowers over each ear. Her white satin gown has a rectangular train. *Vogue*, 10/1/25.

Bride wears *cloche*-style headpiece. Dapper groom wears morning coat (cutaway) with black and gray pin striped trousers, white vest, wing-collar shirt, striped tie, and white spats. *Vogue*, 10/25.

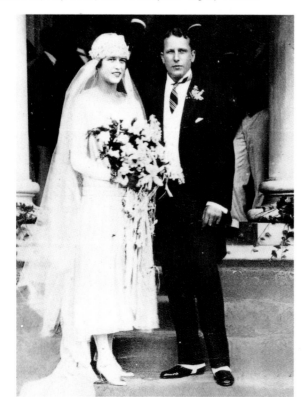

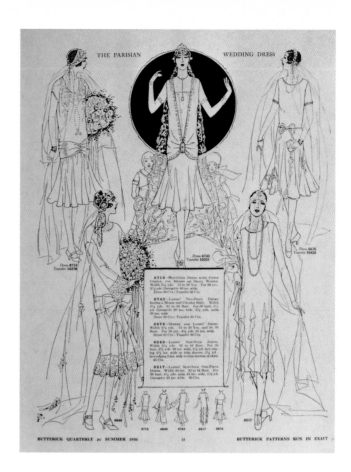

Five wedding gowns—Note: gypsy girdle, circular skirts (three in top row), vertical ruffles (bottom right), and *bandeaux*. *Butterick Quarterly*, 1926. *Courtesy of Rose Jamieson.*

Bride wears wreath of flowers with attached veil, wedding gown adorned with rhinestone baskets containing satin flowers. / Two chiffon attendants dresses accented with chiffon flowers and petals. Stewart & Co., 1925-26.

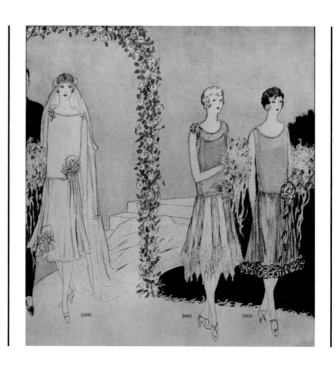

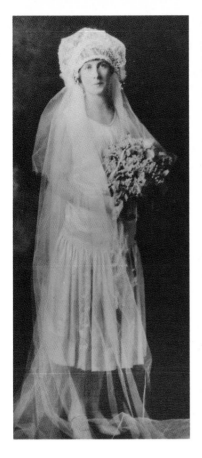
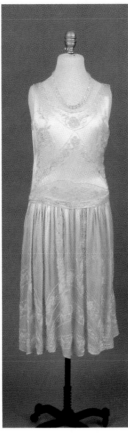
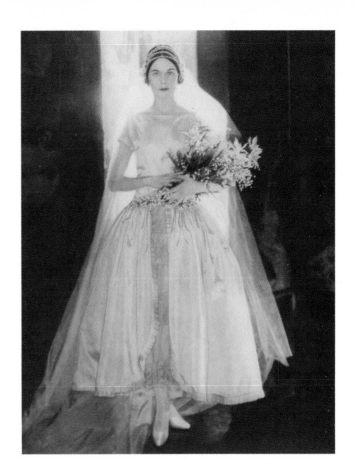

Bride wearing fan-shaped headpiece, white satin gown with dropped waist, 1926. *Courtesy of Jessie E. Ryno.*

White satin wedding dress with crystal seed beads, gathered skirt (similar to gown in previous portrait).

Bride - wears bands of wax buds with attached veil. / Attendant - wears milkmaid-style hat. Both ladies wear dresses with uneven hems and Theo-style shoes with ribbon ties, 8/26. *Courtesy of Louis and Mary Urbanek Manarin.*

Robe de style wedding gown, bouffant taffeta skirt over silver lace, headpiece of flower bands. *Vogue, 4/26. Courtesy of Richard Groman.*

Crepe satin Vionnet gown which is "untrimmed, but with the beauty of cut and line that Vionnet inevitably brings to her creations." *Vogue, 4/26. Courtesy of Richard Groman.*

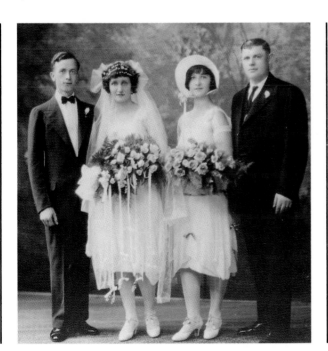

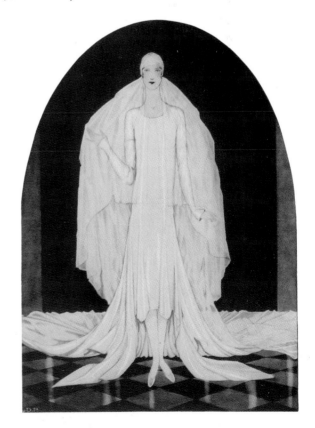

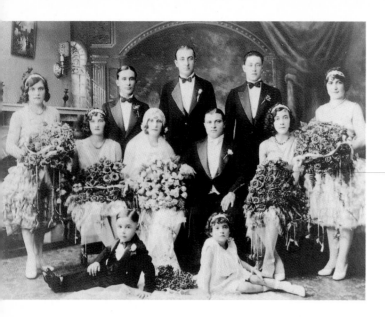

Bride wears a lace veil fastened over her head with cluster of flowers over each ear. Bridesmaids wear headbands and flounced *robe de style* dresses. They carry huge bouquets of four dozen roses each. Groom wears tails, ushers wear tuxedos.

1927

The bias cut (used extensively by designer Madeleine Vionnet) began to grow in popularity. Surplice-style bodices were often paired with layered skirts. The gypsy girdle and the long tied bodice remained in style.

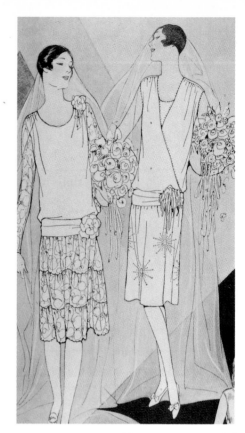

Wedding gowns. / Layered skirt, floral accent. / Surplice bodice, beaded star burst motif. *Pictorial Review*, 1927.

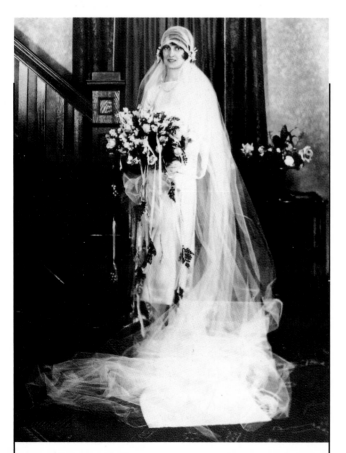

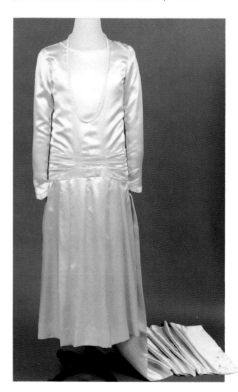

White satin wedding gown with rectangular train from accompanying portrait, 1927. *Courtesy of Kemerer Museum, gift of Lucia Gray.*

Bride wearing veil which is gathered over the head with clusters of orange blossoms over each ear, 1927. *Courtesy of Kemerer Museum, gift of Lucia Gray.*

Late 1928

Bi-level gowns were an unusual option, featuring hemlines which ended at the knee in front and the ankle in the back.

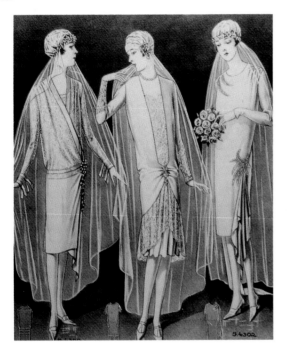

Bridal fashions. Note: surplice bodice, extended bodice, draped skirts. *Reinach's Review of Fashion*, Paris, 1928. *Courtesy of Lehigh County Historical Society.*

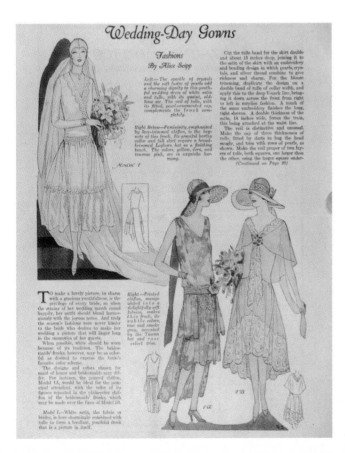

Late 1929

Hemlines dropped to the ankle and waistlines rose to their normal position where they remained throughout the 1930s.

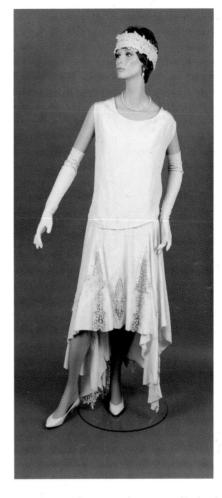

Ivory crepe two-piece wedding gown, lace trimmed bi-level skirt, matching lace *bandeau*, 1929. *Courtesy of Cedar Crest Alumnae Museum, gift of Eloise Howell Sammis.*

Satin wedding gown with deep flounce of tulle, pearl trimmed fitted cap. / Bridesmaids wear garden party hats and bi-level skirts. *Fashion Service*, 1928. *Courtesy of Suzanjoy M. Checksfield.*

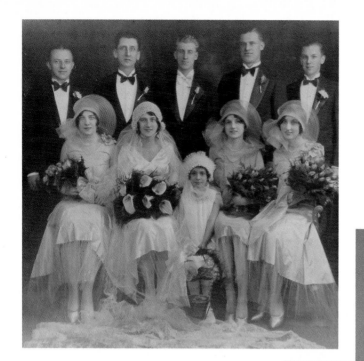

Wedding party of author's mother and father-in-law. Bride holds bouquet of calla lilies, bridesmaids wear horsehair hats and satin gowns with tulle flounces (similar to earlier illustration.) 2/22/30. *Courtesy of Margaretha J Laubner.*

Satin wedding pumps with lily-of-the-valley shoe clips. *Courtesy of Margaretha J. Laubner.*

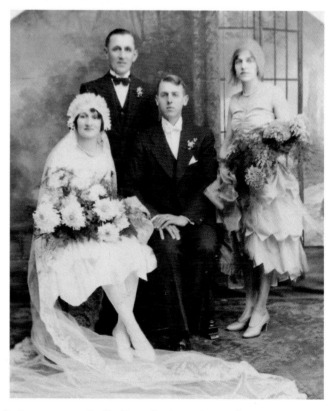

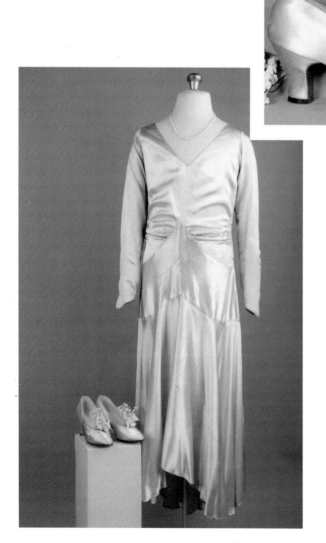

Satin wedding gown, bodice gathered into pointed hip yoke, bias-cut bi-level skirt. Purchased in 1929, worn 2/22/30. *Courtesy of Margaretha J. Laubner.*

Bride wears cap of ruffled lace. Bridesmaid wears "forehead" hat with brim turned up, dress with gathered bodice and layered bi-level skirt. *Courtesy of Roseann Ettinger (Remember When....).*

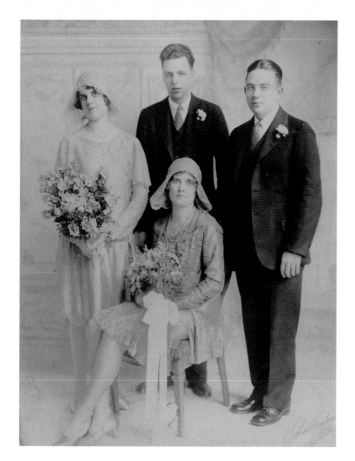

Informal wedding—bride wears short pastel lace dress and helmet-style hat, c. 1928-29.

ATTENDANTS' FROCKS AND GOWNS

Feminine, romantic styles were created for bridal attendants in both long and short lengths. According to *Fashion Service Magazine* of 1928, "When possible, white should be worn [by the bride] because of its tradition. The bridesmaids' frocks, however, may be as colorful as desired to express the bride's favorite color scheme. The designs and colors chosen for the maid of honor and the bridesmaids may differ." Bridesmaids' fashions of soft sheer floral-print fabrics became stylish during the late twenties.

Bride wears long net veil gathered over forehead and trimmed with wax orange blossoms. Groom wears tuxedo fastened with link-button, wing collar, and white bow tie, c. 1920-22.

BRIDAL HEADPIECES

Headpieces were primarily variations of the *cloche*, the *bandeau*, the headband, the coronet, or the fan-effect. It was fashionable, at this time, to decorate headpieces with wax flowers. Small white orange blossoms, with their five pointed petals, were the traditional wedding flower symbolizing chastity and fertility. Attached to the headpiece was a rectangular-shaped veil made of net or lace.

One popular style of head covering was simply a long lace or net veil gathered over the forehead, where it was trimmed with a band of wax orange blossoms.

One, two, or three narrow bands of wax blossoms were placed over the crown of the head or a wreath of blossoms was placed over the forehead.

Wide *bandeaux* (often pointed at the top) were made from white satin or grosgrain ribbon and trimmed with silver embroidery, rhinestones, sequins, crystal beads, or pearls. Pointed lace coronets were also created by fastening lace over a wire frame.

Lace *cloches* often received special treatment over the ears in the form of "lace wheels" or clusters of flowers.

The most unusual headpiece of the period, however, was made of a fan-shaped piece of lace, fastened to the crown of a net or lace cap.

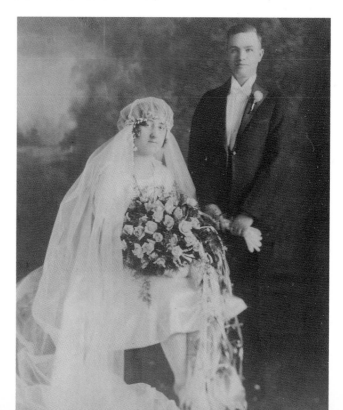

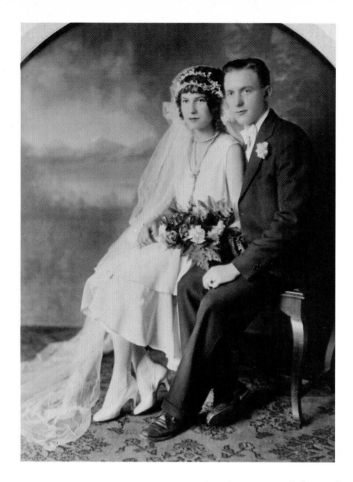

Bride wears double band of wax buds, sleeveless gown with flounced skirt, long knotted strand of pearls, white hose and shoes. c. 1926-30. *Courtesy of Rose Jamieson.*

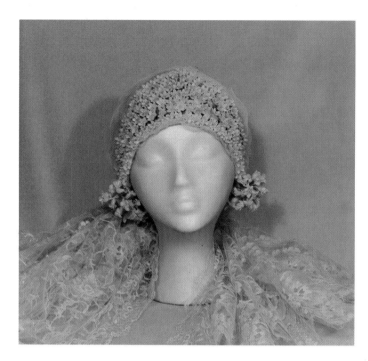

Bridal headpiece (from earlier photo)—wire foundation covered with tulle and wax orange blossoms, clusters of blossoms over each ear, rectangular lace veil. (3 yards long x 2 yards wide). *Courtesy of Margaretha J. Laubner*

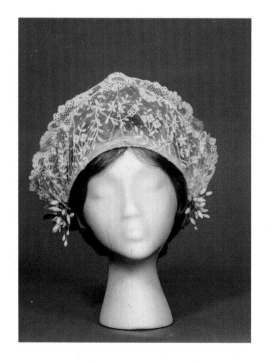

Bridal coronet—lace stretched over a wire foundation with clusters of waxed buds over each ear.

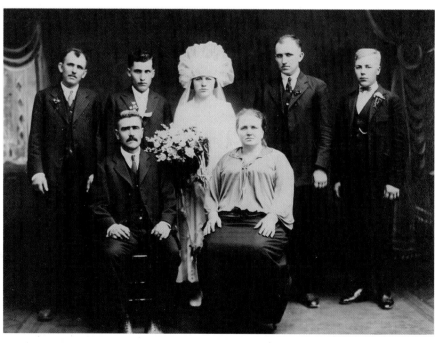

"Jubilant" wedding party—bride wears fan-shaped headpiece, c. 1923-24.

Two views of a fan-shaped headpiece (from earlier photo). Fan supported by wire stays is attached to shirred net cap, four bands of wax buds, 1926. *Courtesy of Cedar Crest Alumnae Museum, gift of Jessie Ryno.*

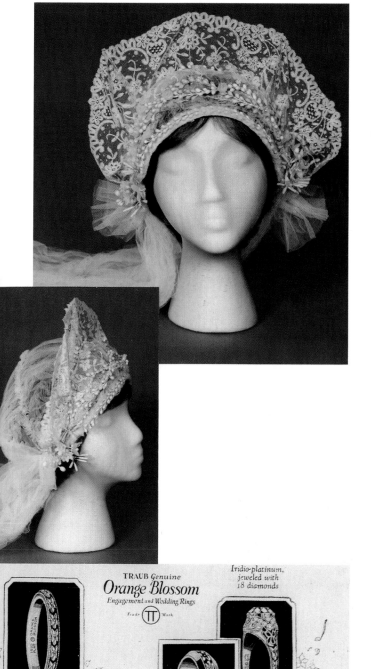

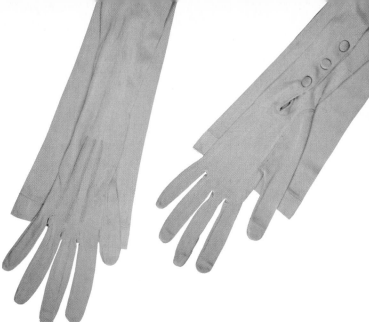

Pale gray silk elbow-length gloves with fabric-covered snaps, worn by bride in 1923. *Courtesy of Cedar Crest Alumnae Museum, gift of Betty Guman.*

ATTENDANTS' HEADPIECES

Wide-brimmed straw or horsehair hats remained in style for bridal attendants throughout the decade. Narrow jeweled headbands or bands of silver laurel leaves were worn over the crown of the head, during the second half of the decade.

BRIDAL BOUQUETS

Bridal bouquets were extremely large, in many cases obscuring the details of the gown. The most common were large round bouquets of roses (often as many as four dozen) accented with a cascade of long white ribbon streamers. Additional flowers and bows were attached to the streamers at varying levels.

Another more sophisticated arrangement featured five or six long stemmed white Calla lilies.

ACCESSORIES

It was customary for the bride to wear a pearl necklace (either long or short) and matching pearl earrings. White gloves, shoes, and stockings completed the ensemble.

Engagement rings and matching wedding bands were introduced in the 1920s. They were often engraved with orange blossoms, forget-me-nots, or wedding bells.

Matching wedding bands and engagement ring with orange blossom motif. *Vogue, 1926. Courtesy of Richard Groman.*

CHAPTER 6:
SPORTSWEAR

With the eight-hour workday, paid vacations, and new time-saving household appliances, liberated women of the 1920s had more leisure time to pursue active or spectator sports. Many of the sportswear designs for women in the twenties were appropriated from men's wear. Knickers, middy blouses, beach pajamas, jodhpurs, vest blouses, Fair Isle or cricket sweaters, lumberjack blouses, and blazers were all adaptations of mens' styles.

"Coco" Chanel was a master at adapting men's wear into casual clothing for women. She is considered by many to be the "creator of modern sportswear for women." Chanel felt that traditional women's garments were too confining for the active women of the twenties. To fill this void in her own wardrobe, she often designed sports clothing for herself. She was an excellent model for these practical garments which attracted the attention of other women who eagerly followed.

Another noted sportswear designer of the 1920s was French *couturier*, Jean Patou. He created attractive wearable sports clothing for his active young clientele. Like Chanel, his trademark was always simplicity of line. He was continually searching for new improved fabrics for his line of sportswear which included fashions for the beach, tennis, golf, and skiing. He was 40 years ahead of his time when he emblazoned his monogram "J.P." on garments from his sportswear line.

The well known tennis player Jane Regny became the first American sportswear designer. She began her career in 1922, designing simple clothing for sports and travel. She is most noted for her wide-leg pants and three-piece bathing ensembles.

Blouses—loose shapeless bodices without darts, wide waistbands trimmed with braid and beading. John Wanamaker, 1921-22.

INFORMAL LEISURE TIME CLOTHING

BLOUSES

Blouses, from the early part of the decade, were quite fancy with necklines similar to those on dresses of the period. They were made of soft fabrics such as georgette and crepe de chine. Embroidery, beading, braid, and lace were the principle forms of ornamentation.

By the second half of the decade, blouses had a more tailored masculine appearance and were often worn with a four-in-hand tie. Long overblouses were banded at the hip, or were belted over the blouse at the natural waist.

Green rayon knit blouse—boat-neck, bell sleeves, wide waistband, bodice trimmed with seed beads. / Brown and green pleated wool skirt. Note: resemblance to previous blouse illustrations. *Courtesy of Cedar Crest Alumnae Museum, gift of Miriam Woodring Alexander.*

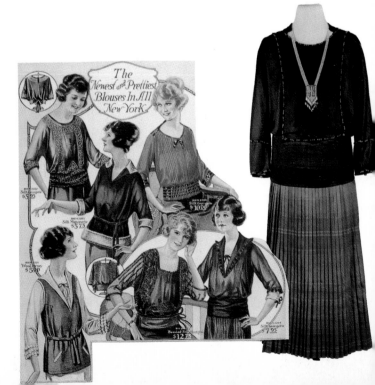

Middy Blouse

The middy blouse, a carry-over from the preceding decades, was patterned after the enlisted man's sailor uniform. The breast pocket, sailor collar, and long sleeves were decorated with nautical emblems, service stripes, and braided trim. They were made of white cotton or linen for summer; and black, navy, or red wool serge or flannel for winter. A contrasting silk or poplin tie was knotted or slipped through a loop at the base of the collar. Middy blouses were worn with skirts or with knickers for sport. They were also worn with black wool bloomers for school gym classes.

White cotton twill middy blouse with sailor collar, black silk necktie. Label: Patria. / Heavy black wool gym bloomers. *Courtesy of Cedar Crest Alumnae Museum, gift of Ellie Laubner.* / Rubber sole canvas shoes with buttoned straps.

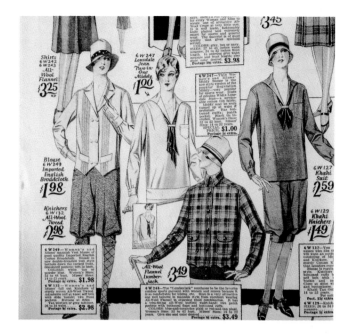

Cotton tucked vest blouse, wool tweed knickers, knicker socks. / Cotton jean middy blouse. / Wool flannel lumberjack blouse. / Khaki knicker suit. National Cloak and Suit Co., 1927.

Lumberjack Blouse

The masculine lumberjack blouse was made of wool plaid with a pointed or knitted collar, patch pockets, and banded waist. It was often worn with knickers.

A-lumberjack sweater; C, D, E, G, J-cardigans; B, F, H-coat sweaters; K-Jacquard cricket sweater. Sears, Roebuck and Co., 1928-29.

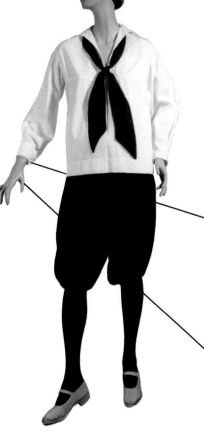

Vest Blouse

The popular man-tailored vest blouse had long or short sleeves, a notched collar, and a pointed cutaway-style hem (resembling a man's vest). These blouses were worn outside of the skirt or knickers.

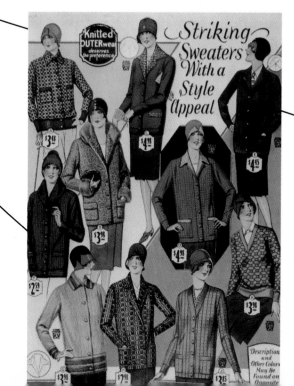

SWEATERS

Coat Sweater

In the early teens, Chanel responded to her need for casual clothing by creating a heavy tricot sweater which she patterned after those worn by Normandy fishermen. Tricot was previously considered a lowly fabric, suitable only for undergarments. These "coat" sweaters, as they were later called, had high shawl collars and crisscross-style belts. There was little change in the styling of these sweaters from the teens to the late 1920s.

Fair Isle

The Scottish Fair Isle sweater experienced immediate and continuing success after its introduction by the Prince of Wales (later Duke of Windsor) in 1922. It was made in the V-neck pullover style and featured colorful patterned stripes. It was often referred to as a "cricket" sweater in mail-order catalogs of the period.

Cubist Style

Jean Patou and Jane Regny are remembered for their Cubist style sweaters, which were inspired by the abstract paintings of Sonia Delaunay and Piet Mondrian. They featured bold geometric shapes in attractive eye catching colors.

Trompe L'oeil

Italian designer, Elsa Schiaparelli, moved to Paris in 1928. She loved to shock and amuse people with her witty designs. She began her career by designing black hand-knit sweaters with a white ribbon bow knitted into the neck. The bow was designed to give the illusion of three dimensions; but was, in reality, just an illustration knitted into the flat surface of the sweater. These were known as her "*trompe l'oeil*" sweaters, which means "trick of the eye" in French.

Lustrous pink rayon cardigan sweater with buttoned sash. / Oriental-style paper parasol with wooden ribs. *Courtesy of Gladys Marhefka.*

BLAZERS

Handy blazer style jackets for women were introduced in the 1920s. They were often made of striped cotton or flannel and were produced in a variety of colors.

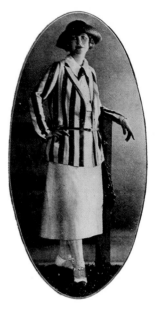

Striped flannel blazer with narrow belt by Spalding, available in a variety of colors. *Town & Country*, 8/22. *Courtesy of Judy Carpenter.*

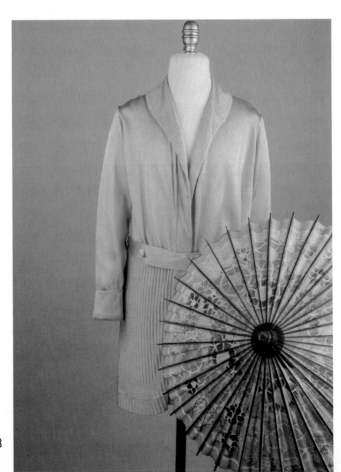

SKIRTS

In the early twenties, long narrow barrel-shaped skirts reached just below the calf. Serge, khaki, silk, poplin, and satin were the common fabrics. Short knife and box pleated skirts were prevalent after 1925. In 1929, accordion pleated skirts were offered in leading mail-order catalogs.

KNICKERS

Serge or tweed knickers were worn for general sportswear and hiking. They were fastened with buttons at the waist and the knee bands.

Knickers were worn with cotton or wool "knicker" socks in neutral shades of brown, tan, blue, and gray. They were often made with striped or "pineapple" (diamond-shaped) ribs. The turnovers (cuffs) were often decorated with geometric designs or Argyle patterns. (It is a popular belief that the Argyle pattern originated from the Scottish tartan of the Duke of Argyle.)

Cotton Argyle knicker socks. *Courtesy of Suzanjoy M. Checksfield.* / Heavy brown wool knickers, self belt, two-buttoned plackets, buttoned knee bands.

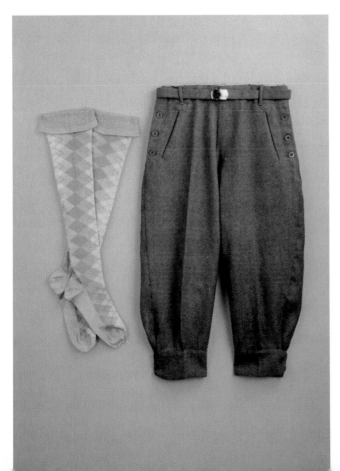

BATHING AND BASKING

Until the 1920s, suntanned skin was the occupational hazard of peasant workers, to be avoided at all costs by gentle folk. Ladies went to great lengths to protect their lily white skin by the use of wide-brimmed hats and parasols.

When Chanel returned from the French Riviera with a tan, she established a new vogue for golden brown skin. An off-season tan then became a status symbol, indicating that the individual had the means and the leisure time to travel to warmer climes during the harsh winter months. Tanning was such a novelty, I was told by a former flapper, that before basking in the sun, she and her friends would spell their initials on their arms with strips of adhesive tape, just to see the amazing results when the tape was removed.

The new mobility created by modern modes of transportation, made it possible for many people of moderate means to leave the cities for a day or a weekend at the seaside.

BATHING SUITS

Dressmaker Bathing Suit

The dressmaker suit consisted of a sleeveless V-neck tunic with matching shorts and sash. They were made of woven fabrics such as satin, taffeta, or printed broad cloth, and were often trimmed with white piping.

Gray wool one-piece bathing suit, trunks attached at waist. Label: Piqua Hosiery Co. *Courtesy of Richard Groman.*

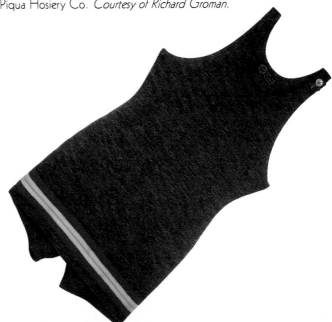

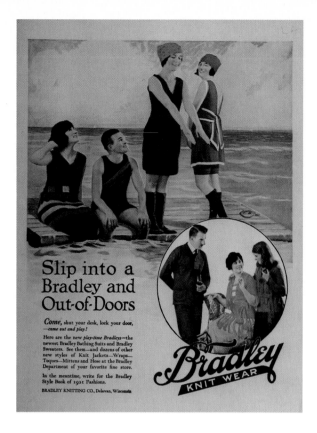

Loose-fitting knitted bathing suits and sweaters by Bradley Knit wear, 1921.

Aviator-style rubber bathing cap. / California-style one-piece red worsted bathing suit, trunks attached at waist. / Rubber bathing slippers. All available in red, green, and blue. National Cloak and Suit Co., 1928. *Courtesy of Suzanjoy M. Checksfield.*

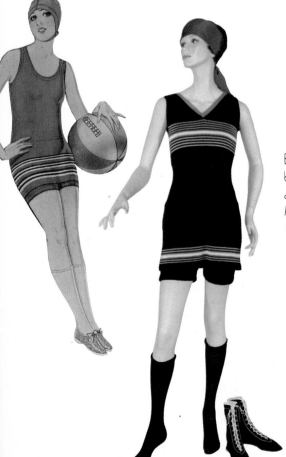

Black wool knit one-piece bathing suit, trunks attached at waist. Label: Gantner & Mattern Co., San Francisco. *Courtesy of Jean Weaber.*

California-Style Knitted Bathing Suit

According to *Time and Life,* flappers wearing the new one-piece California-style bathing suit were carried off the beaches in 1922 for indecent exposure. This "daring" new wool knit suit consisted of a form-fitting hip-length tank top with matching trunks which were attached at the waist. Common colors for these suits were red, blue, black, gray, and kelly green with contrasting stripes. This "risqué" suit became commonplace by 1924.

Leotard Bathing Suit

A third style of suit, introduced in the late twenties, consisted of a sleeveless V-neck leotard worn under contrasting belted trunks.

By 1929, low-cut "sunback" bathing suits were advertised in fashion catalogs.

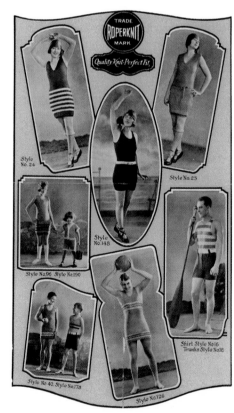

Knit bathing suits for men, women, and children by Roper. Note: *bandeaux,* belts, rolled hose, laced beach shoes. c. 1925-30.

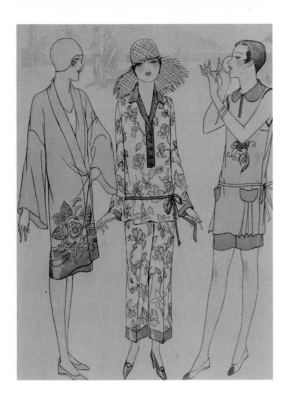

Beachwear—Chinese coolie coat. / Chinese beach pajamas. / Dressmaker two-piece bathing suit. *McCall Quarterly*, summer 1927.

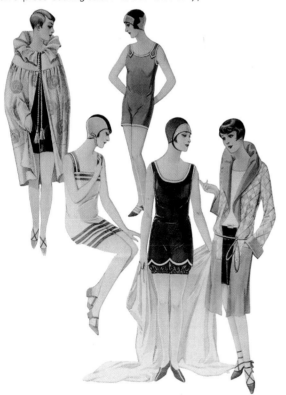

Beach attire. / Terry cloth bathing cloak with Pierrot collar. / Two tricot suits. / Black taffeta suit. / Terry cloth beach coat. / Aviator caps. *Reinach's Review of Fashion*, Paris, 1928. *Courtesy of Lehigh County Historical Society, Pennsylvania.*

Advertising fan—flapper wearing head scarf tied in the manner worn by 1920s bathers.

BEACH PAJAMAS

Chanel also introduced beach pajamas which consisted of a belted tunic and wide leg "gob" pants (slang for sailor pants—later called bell-bottoms). They were made of silk, crepe de chine, and cotton, and their wide legs gave the appearance of a long skirt.

COOLIE COATS

The thigh-length Chinese-style coolie coat was often worn as a beach cover-up over the bathing suit. They were made of silk, crepe de chine, and cotton and were produced in Oriental floral and bamboo prints.

BATHING CLOAKS

Bathing cloaks, which often featured a ruffled "Pierrot" collar, were also popular. They were made of silk, sateen, or challis.

HEADGEAR

Women wore some form of head covering on the beach which included a triangular silk head scarf, a rubber bandanna, or gum rubber "diving cap" (with or without the aviator-style chin strap).

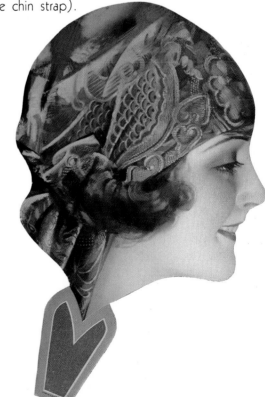

BEACH SHOES

High-cut canvas beach shoes which laced up the front were a carry-over from the teens, but could still be seen on the beaches as late as 1927. The new short "sand tight" gum-rubber swimming shoes were also available in red, green, blue, and black. The Franklin Simon & Co. advertised a pair of satin bathing shoes in its 1926 catalog. Bathing shoes were worn with black cotton stockings which were rolled down below the knees.

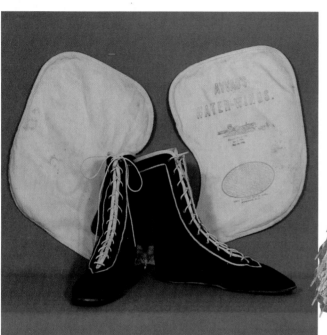

Black canvas beach shoes with white piping, binding, and laces; thin white rubber soles. / Ayvad cotton "water wings" (inflatable floatation device).

PARASOLS

Parasols were used by those who did not wish to acquire a tan or those who had had too much sun. Short inexpensive Oriental-style parasols were all the rage in the late 1920s. They contained 30-36 protruding wooden ribs and a thick wooden handle. These styles generally had cotton or paper covers decorated with Oriental designs. Due to the growing popularity of sun tanning, however, the parasol was headed toward extinction.

GOLF

Women golfers wore tailored dresses or sweaters with pleated skirts. They were made of a variety of fabrics from wool to washable silk. Comfortable brogues, kiltie oxfords, or saddle shoes were worn with striped or pineapple ribbed hose.

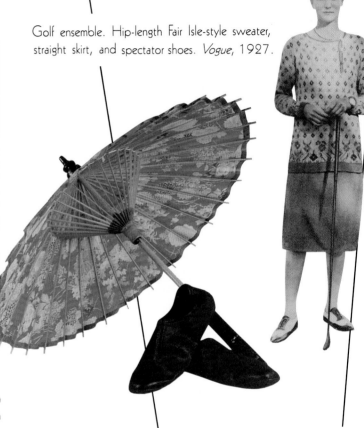

Golf ensemble. Hip-length Fair Isle-style sweater, straight skirt, and spectator shoes. *Vogue*, 1927.

Short stocky Oriental-style parasol—floral print cotton cover, thirty wooden ribs, thick wooden handle. / Black rubber bathing slippers. *Courtesy of Cedar Crest Alumnae Museum, gift of Marion Kingsbury.*

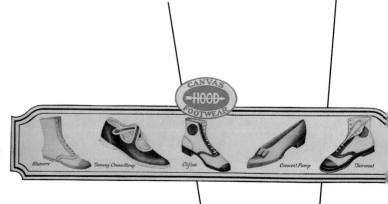

Canvas sport shoes by Hood, 1920.

TENNIS

Mlle. Suzanne Lenglen, French six-time Wimbledon champion (1919 to 1926), modernized the women's tennis costume by eliminating the traditional corset, petticoats, long skirt, and man-tailored blouse. In their place she simply wore a white calf-length jumper, colorful *bandeau*, and white rolled down hose. For cooler weather, a colorful fur trimmed cardigan sweater was added. Her ensembles, on and off the court, were designed by renowned French *couturier*, Jean Patou. His attractive ensembles set the example for modern sportswomen around the world.

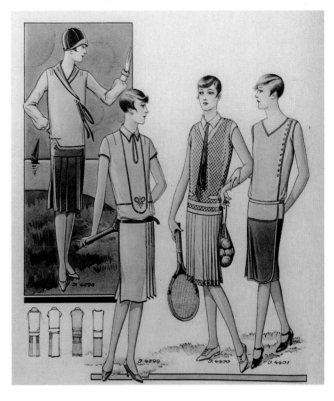

Tennis frocks of stockinette, crepe de chine, and rayon in red, white, and blue. Note: Eton crop hair styles. *Reinach's Review of Fashion*, Paris, 1928. *Courtesy of Lehigh County Historical Society, Pennsylvania.*

Tennis trend setter Suzanne Lenglen - white jumper, *bandeau*, and white rolled-down hose. *Town & Country* magazine, 8/22. *Courtesy of Judy Carpenter.*

SKIING

A heavy woolen coat sweater or lumberjack-style jacket was worn with woolen knickers and heavy knicker socks. A knitted scarf, gloves, and hat with a large pompon completed the look.

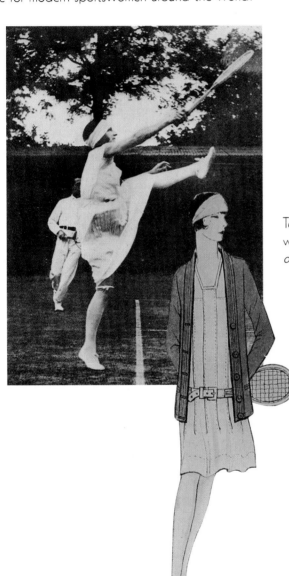

Tennis outfit (à la Suzanne Lenglen). Knee-length white cotton or silk tennis jumper, colorful jersey cardigan, white silk *bandeau*, white hose, and saddle shoes. *Modern Priscilla* magazine, 1928.

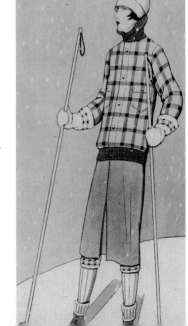

Ski ensemble—knit hat, lumberjack jacket, skirt with inverted pleat (knickers were the norm), gauntlet-style mittens, knicker socks. *Vogue*, 1/25. *Courtesy of Richard Groman.*

HORSEBACK RIDING

The informal sidesaddle riding habit included a hacking jacket, a calf-length wraparound riding skirt, a white man-tailored shirt, and a four-in-hand tie. A "vagabond," "knockabout," or Derby hat; and riding boots completed the ensemble.

The Sears, Roebuck and Co. catalogs from 1921 through 1923 featured riding habits of khaki cloth. They consisted of long loose knee-length belted riding coats (similar to suit jackets of the period). They were advertised with breeches which were "finished off at the bottom with eyelets and fastened with laces."

Originally from India, jodhpurs were first worn by Western men circa the First World War. The 1926 Franklin Simon & Co. women's catalog offered riding habits which included jodhpurs (flared from the hip to the knee, and tight from knee to the ankle); a long sleeveless whipcord vest or beltless hacking jacket (flared from the waist to accommodate the jodhpurs); a white man-tailored blouse; a four-in-hand tie; leather riding boots; and a knockabout, vagabond, or Derby hat.

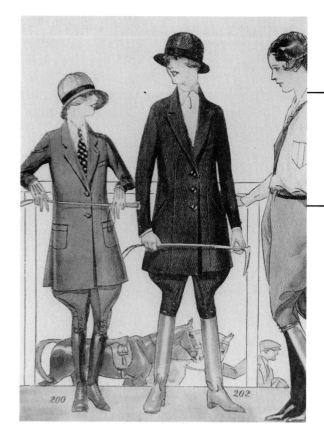

Girls' riding habits—coats and breeches of gabardine, melton, English tweed, or whipcord. Milan straw knockabout hats. Franklin Simon & Co., 1926. *Courtesy of Kemerer Museum, gift of Barbara Stout.*

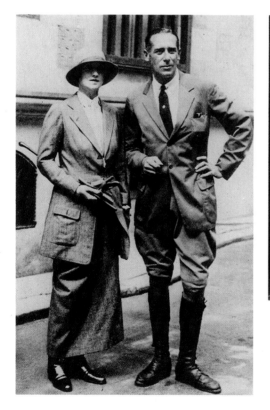

Informal sidesaddle riding habit with knockabout hat. *Town & Country*, 1922. *Courtesy of Judy Carpenter.*

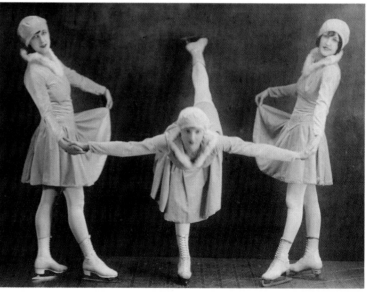

The "European Girl Trio"—short velvet figure skating dresses with white fur trim, matching berets and tights, c. 1923.

CHAPTER 7:
OUTERWEAR

CLOTH COATS

Coats commonly take their lead from the dress silhouette of any given period, and the 1920s were no exception.

1920-1922

Long oversized coats reached below the calf, completely enveloping the body, which was a carry-over from the teens. Their shapeless bodices and slightly flared skirts created large wedge-shaped silhouettes. These coats had high-waisted self-fabric belts which often crisscrossed and buttoned in front. The set-in sleeves had deep cuffs.

The broad cape-like collars (when opened), converted to high-standing "choker" collars, which completely encircled the throat (when closed). They were trimmed with coney, opossum, beaver, raccoon, rabbit, Manchurian wolf, squirrel, novelty monkey fur, and skunk. Less expensive synthetic fur was also available. Coats were often accented with ornamental buttons and an occasional tassel or two. Jackets were merely shortened versions of the coat styles.

Straight-line surplice-style coats—shawl collars, top coat with batwing sleeves, and two coats with bell-style sleeves, arrowhead stitching. *Elite Styles*, 1923.

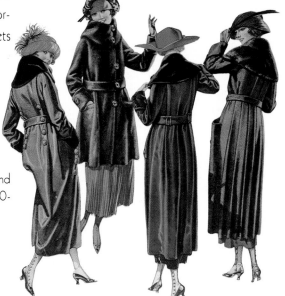

Roomy high-waisted coats of velveteen plush, "beaver fur cloth," and wool; large convertible cape-like collars. Montgomery Ward, 1920-21.

1923-1924

Roomy straight-line surplice-style coats were fastened with one large "platter button" over the right hip. Shawl collars, cuffs, and hems continued to be trimmed with fur. The most common sleeves were the batwing and the bell sleeve. Top stitching and embroidery were popular forms of ornamentation, and arrows were a favorite motif.

1925-1926

Short knee-length coats often contained godets at the hem, which created a slight flare. Double-breasted coats were made with notched or shawl collars.

Surplice-style coats featured wide pointed collars, formed by the combination of the collar and the lapel. They were often faced with a contrasting color, or the collar portion was trimmed with fur. The back portion of the collar was normally worn up. When buttoned, it converted to a high "mushroom" collar.

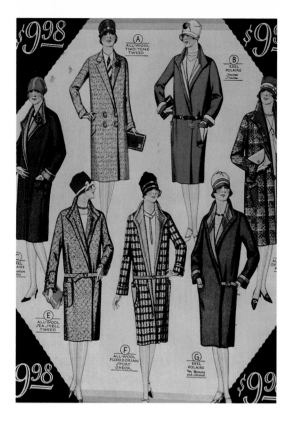

Tubular double-breasted, surplice, and edge-to-edge front fastening coats—notched and pointed collars, hip belts. National Coat & Suit Co., 1927.

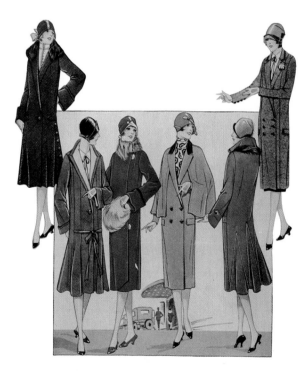

Knee-length coats—straight-line and flared skirts; pointed, mushroom, and notched collars. *Pictorial Review*, 10/25.

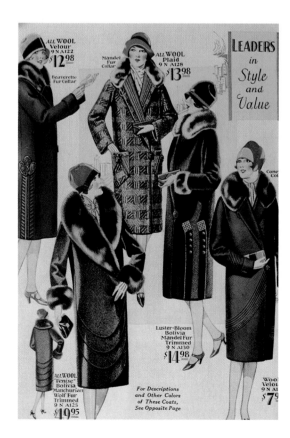

Tubular surplice-style coats—mushroom and shawl collars, decorative parallel top stitching. Charles William Stores, winter 1927-28.

Coats became slender tubes enhanced with top-stitch-ing, tucks, or seams in Art Deco-style radiating sunbursts, converging diagonals, and sweeping parallel lines. Self or contrasting belts, and decorative fabric *boutonnières* were often included.

Coats were made of wool, vicuña, velveteen plush, wool velour, silk seal plush, and astrakhan cloth (resembling Persian lamb). Brown, tan, rust, cranberry, gray, black, and gracklehead blue (medium blue) were the most popular colors.

Luxurious fur coats were created from sable, mink, caracul, beaver, Hudson seal, civet cat, mole, squirrel, dyed rabbit, and nutria. They were generally made in the surplice style.

French designer Jacques Heim began his career in 1923, when he took over the family fur business. This firm was noted for its chic high-fashion fur coats.

The American firm of H. Jaekel and Sons maintained a showroom on New York's Fifth Avenue. House designers created sumptuous fur coats with distinctive design and ex-cellent tailoring. Also featured were cloth coats enriched with luxurious fur trim.

Raccoon coats were popular with college students, es-pecially for football games and rides in open roadsters. They were mid-calf or slightly longer, with a large shawl collar and deep cuffs. The pelts were usually arranged to form four horizontal stripes at the bottom.

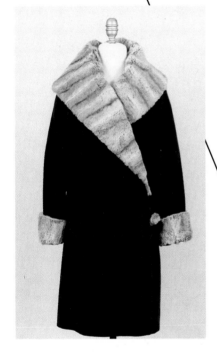

Knee-length surplice-style coat of blue velveteen plush, squirrel collar and cuffs, c. 1926-30. *Courtesy of Kemerer Museum, gift of Mrs. Edmund Martin.*

Raccoon coat with large shawl collar, four large celluloid buttons, pat-terned rayon satin lining, c. 1925.

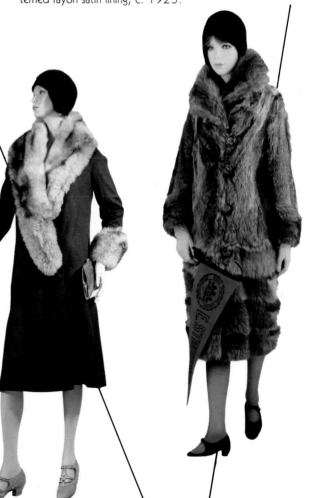

Dark green wool coat with surplice closing, (possibly) beaver fur collar and cuffs. Label: May's, N.Y.

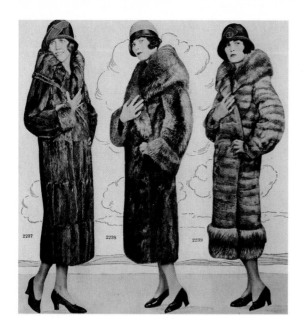

Fur coats of muskrat, opossum, and muskrat with dyed blue fox fur collar and border. Stewart & Co., 1925-26.

EVENING WRAPS AND COATS

Early evening capes and wraps with dolman, batwing, and kimono sleeves were reminiscent of the exotic designs of Paul Poiret. Common fabrics were silk, velvet, satin, lamé, and gold and silver brocades. They were decorated with embroidery, metallic braids, tassels, or bands of fur. These designs often incorporated high shirred or fur trimmed collars. Popular colors were black, sapphire, jade, and raspberry.

During the second half of the decade, short fitted coats were worn with enormous fur collars and cuffs. Opulent designer coats were highlighted by metallic braids, embroidery, and glittering *diamanté*.

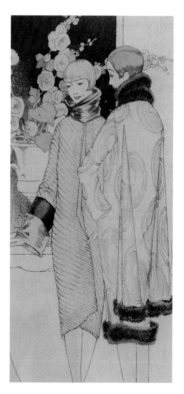

Fur evening coats - /Winter ermine with white fox collar, by Heim, Paris. / Large-collared cape with diagonally styled white fitch pelts, by Grunwaldt, Paris. *Ladies' Home Journal*, 10/28.

Evening wraps. / Quilted lamé banded in black satin. / Gray and silver brocade, banded in kolinsky, by French designer Lucien Lelong. *Ladies' Home Journal*, 11/25.

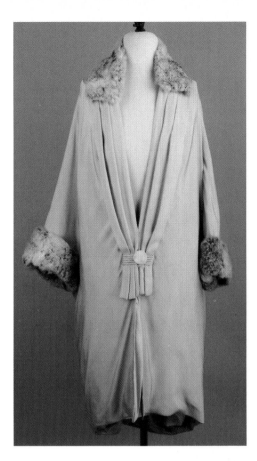

Front view—almond silk crepe dolman with deep V edge-to-edge closing and rabbit fur trim. Purchased in Paris, 1926. Label: Gimbel Brothers, Paris. *Courtesy of Richard Groman.*

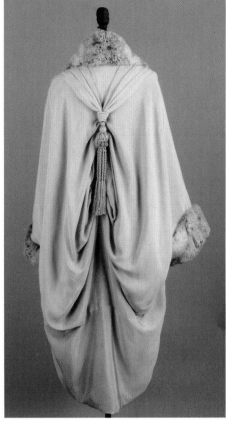

Back view—wonderfully draped with exotic silk cord tassel.

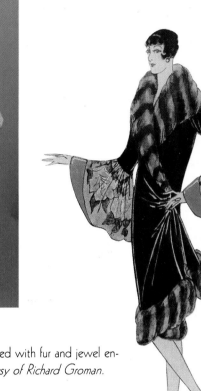

Chic evening wrap of patterned lamé trimmed with fur and jewel encrusted embroidery. *Vogue,* 9/26. *Courtesy of Richard Groman.*

Black velvet evening coat with flowered lamé sleeves and fur trim, by Lucile, Paris. *McCall's,* 2/27.

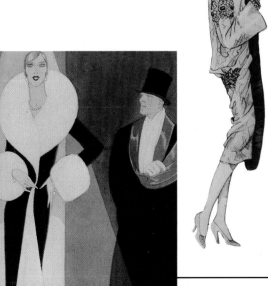

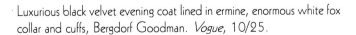

Luxurious black velvet evening coat lined in ermine, enormous white fox collar and cuffs, Bergdorf Goodman. *Vogue,* 10/25.

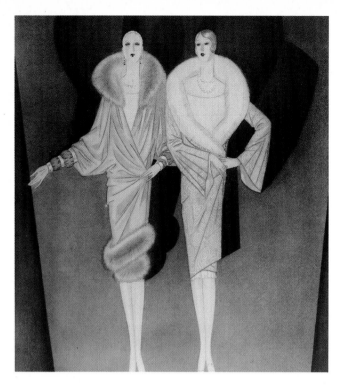

Fur trimmed evening coats with dolman and bell sleeves. *Vogue*, 3/27. Courtesy of Richard Groman.

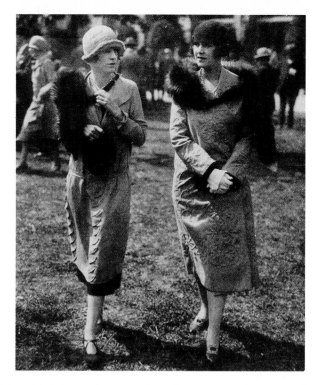

Fashionable ladies at the races wearing fur pieces over their coats. *Town & Country*, 6/25. Courtesy of Judy Carpenter.

FUR PIECES

Fur pieces, also called "fur scarves," were an important status symbol worn throughout the 1920s and 1930s. The entire animal came complete with legs, a tail, and a head featuring beady glass eyes and a spring tension mouth. Furs were nonchalantly draped over the shoulders of a dress or suit. They could then be fastened by snapping two of the feet together or by squeezing the clothespin-style mouth to make the animal grip its leg.

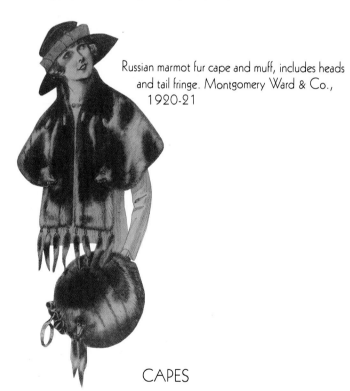

Russian marmot fur cape and muff, includes heads and tail fringe. Montgomery Ward & Co., 1920-21

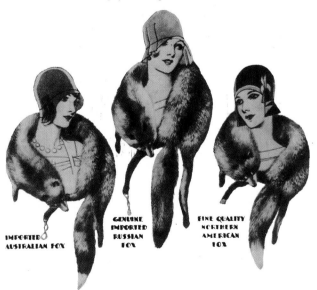

Fox fur pieces. Sears, Roebuck & Co., 1928-29.

CAPES

During the early twenties, stylish fur capes were trimmed along the edges, using animal tails as fringe. Matching muffs containing an animal's head, paws, and tail were also popular. These styles were a carry-over from the teens and soon went out of fashion. Cloth capes played a limited role as part of a matching ensemble or they were attached to the shoulders of a suit or coat.

SHAWLS AND STOLES

Square Spanish-style silk shawls were beautifully embroidered with colorful flowers and edged with silk *macramé* fringe. A few of the popular colors were white, pink, peach, jade, flame, and black. They were often worn with *robe de style* gowns introduced by Jeanne Lanvin. Many people, however, preferred to drape these attractive shawls over their grand pianos, thus the name "piano shawl." Less expensive versions could also be purchased in rayon.

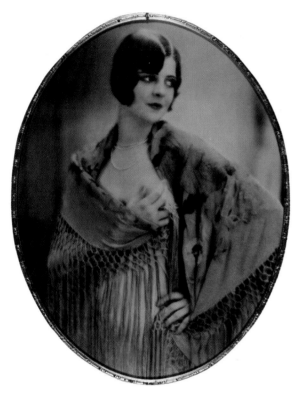

Flapper wrapped in colorful silk shawl with *macramé* fringe. *Courtesy of Mary Anne Faust (Yesterday's Delights).*

As a result of the excitement surrounding the discovery of King Tut's tomb, exotic linen stoles were imported from Egypt. They were referred to as *"Assuit"* stoles, named after the Egyptian city in which they have been made from ancient times to the present day. Due to the difficulties in translation from the Arabic alphabet, the word *Assuit* has been spelled in many ways. I am told that the spelling which provides the most accurate sounds in the English language is *Assuit.*

These rectangular stoles were made of loosely woven linen net (typically white). They were then decorated by hand with millions of shiny pieces of metal fastened to the stole in decorative motifs. During the 1920s, the metal pieces were arranged in geometric patterns, a reflection of the Art Deco movement. The motion of the body caused these stoles to shimmer, as each tiny metal piece reflected the light.

Square white silk shawl embroidered with polychromatic silk thread, trimmed with white silk *macramé* fringe. *Courtesy of Kemerer Museum, gift of Mrs. Byron C. Hayes.*

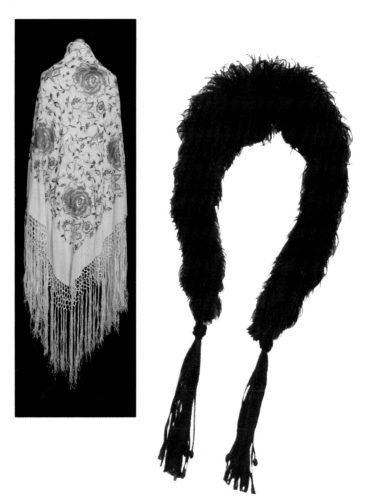

Fluffy black ostrich feather boa with black silk tassels.

BOAS

Short ostrich feather boas with long silk tassels (a carryover from the teens) were worn through the first half of the decade. Popular colors were black, white, navy, gray, and brown.

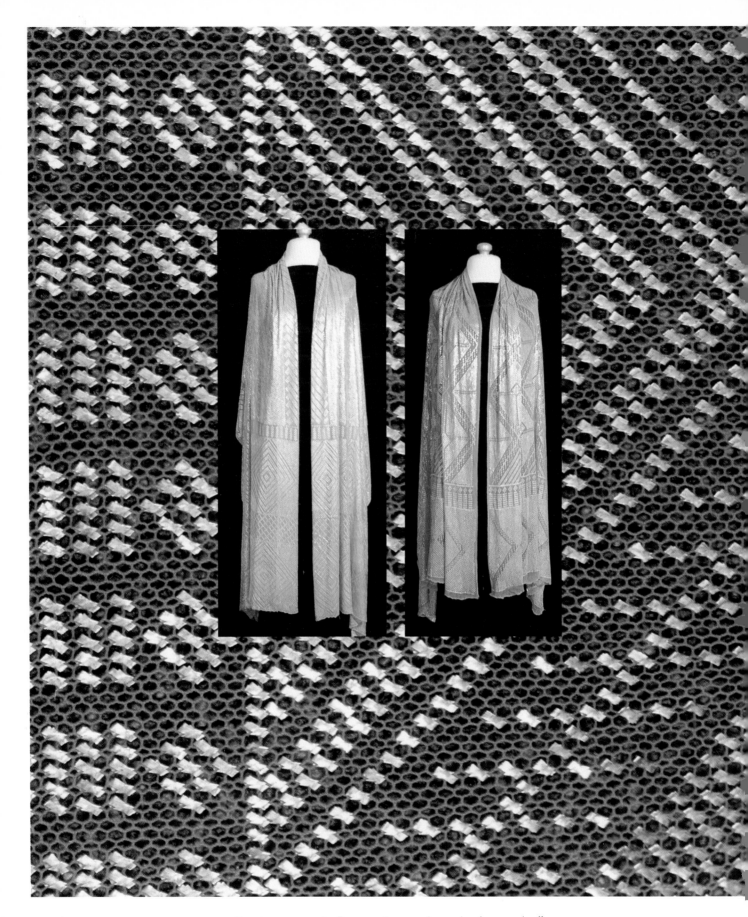

Two large rectangular Egyptian Assuit stoles made of rust and saffron colored linen mesh and hand decorated with millions of tiny shimmering pieces of metal in geometric Art Deco motifs. *Courtesy of The Kemerer Museum, gift of Nina Mackall.*

CHAPTER 8
HAIR AND HEADGEAR

HAIR STYLES

Women had been wearing their hair long since the dawn of time, styling it according to the dictates of fashion. During the teens, women pulled their hair into large Grecian-style chignons at the back of the head. Teenage girls wore their hair in long bouncy ringlets or pulled back with a large bow at the nape of the neck.

EARPHONES

In the first few years of the decade, it was fashionable to wear the hair in curious coiled buns projecting from the ears. These were affectionately called "earphones" or "cootie garages."

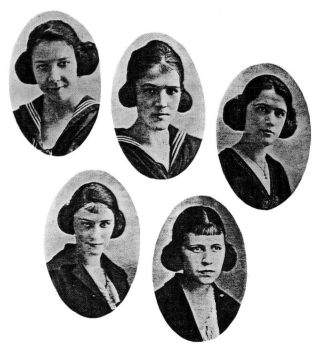

Coeds wearing the "earphones" hair style, from the East Stroudsburg State Teachers' College yearbook, 1921. *Courtesy of East Stroudsburg University.*

THE BOB

Shortly before World War I, the celebrated ballroom dancer Irene Castle introduced a radical new short hair style called the bob. This style was simply a blunt cut, level with the bottom of the ears all around the head. It was worn either with bangs or with the hair brushed off of the forehead. By 1921, following the lead of fashion designer "Coco" Chanel and actresses Clara Bow and Louise Brooks, young women everywhere took the plunge and bobbed their hair. Many women felt compelled to cut their hair in order to accommodate the popular new head-hugging *cloche*-style hats. Since the cutting of hair was still a male-dominated occupation, most young girls had their first bob at a barber shop.

Short hair, along with shorter skirts, soon became a fashion statement and a symbol of women's struggle for independence and equality with men. In 1920, F. Scott Fitzgerald, the popular American novelist, recorded for posterity the trials and tribulations of short hair in his novel *Bernice Bobs Her Hair.*

SHINGLE

As hair dressers became more skilled at their craft, other more sophisticated cuts were introduced. The shingle or "boyish bob," introduced in 1923, featured hair which tapered to a V at the nape of the neck, with either waves or "spit curls" at the sides.

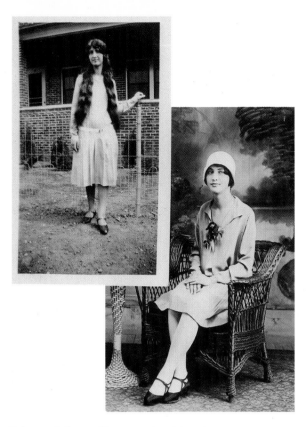

MARCEL WAVE

In 1872, a poor French hairstylist named Marcel Grateau discovered that by grasping the hair with a heated curling iron and flipping it upside down, he could produce natural looking waves. The "Marcel wave," as it was eventually called, reached the height of its popularity during the 1920s and early 1930s. Early curling irons or double-wave crimping irons were heated over the flames of the gas stove, which often left a messy black carbon residue on the iron. Old newspaper or wet fingers were used to gage the temperature. In addition to these early irons, the 1920 Montgomery Ward catalog advertised the modern spring tension electric curling iron which plugged conveniently into any light socket. These irons could maintain the correct temperature and produce "beautiful luxuriant waves" in only five minutes.

Before and after—/ Teenage girl with long hair of the late teens. / Same girl with bobbed hair, early 20s. *Courtesy of Rose Jamieson.*

ETON CROP

The most severe of the short hair styles was the "Eton crop," which appeared in 1926. The hair was shingled all around the head exposing the ears. This style gave new meaning to the word short, as it was patterned after the mandatory hair style for boys at the prestigious Eton preparatory school near London. For the do-it-yourselfer wishing to save the price of a haircut, the hair clipper/neck shaver was available.

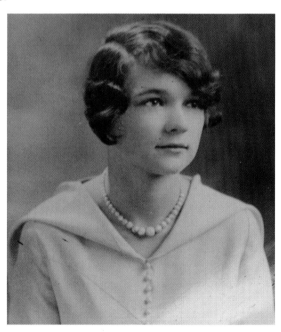

The author's mother Elizabeth in 1928, wearing shingled hair with finger waves ending in Spanish-style "spit curls" over the cheeks. *Courtesy of Elizabeth Pascoe Whitfield.*

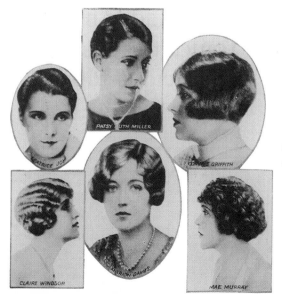

Movie stars wearing the latest hair styles. / Top row—two Eton crops, one shingle hair style. / Bottom row—three bobbed hair styles. *McCall's,* 2/27.

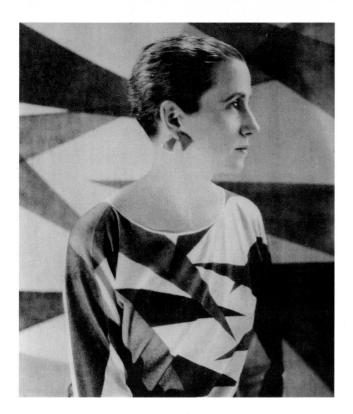

"Madame Agnès, the famous French milliner, is a perfect example of the great chic to be found in modernistic art as applied to costume," *Vogue*, 10/25. Note: Eton crop hair style.

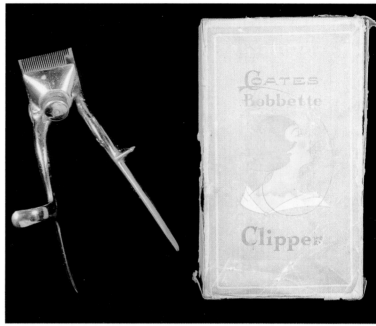

Coates Bobbette hair clipper for shaving the neck. *Courtesy of Rose Jamieson.*

WATER WAVE COMBS AND WAVERS

Waves could also be created (while the hair was wet) with a set of six to eight "water wave combs." A comb was placed approximately an inch below the part. The comb was then used to push the hair upward causing it to curve into a partial wave. The comb was left in the hair and the process was repeated at one inch intervals for the desired number of waves. The combs were then held in place by wrapping ribbon, string, or a scarf around the head until the hair was dry.

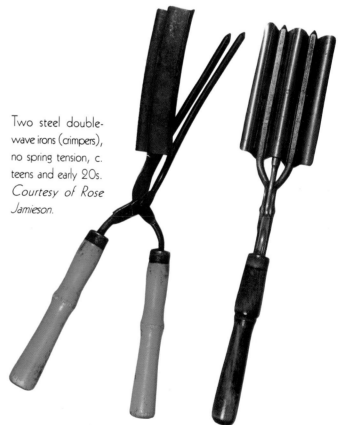

Two steel double-wave irons (crimpers), no spring tension, c. teens and early 20s. *Courtesy of Rose Jamieson.*

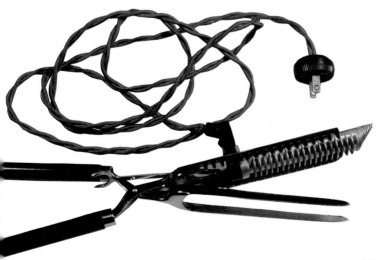

The SUBPEDO waver used by professional French hairdressers. Place the fork side under the hair, close, then draw the ridged cylindrical heating element back using the thumb lever to create the "perfect marcelling". Marked: Marcel Wave Co. Pat 1920.

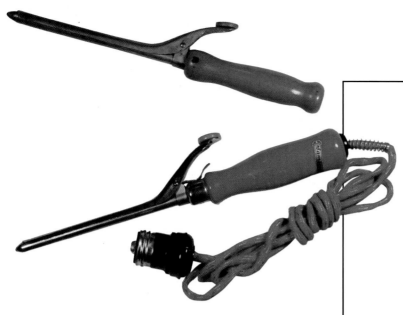

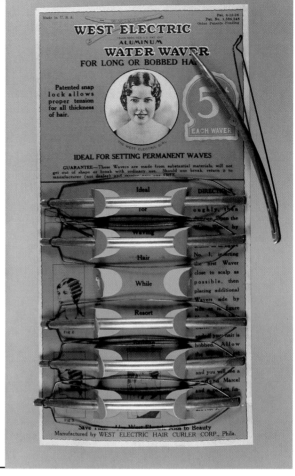

Curling irons. / Steel curling iron with spring tension and thumb rest. *Courtesy of Rose Jamieson.* / Electric version of same curling iron, plug screwed into light socket. Marked: Samson, Arrow - H&H U.S.A.

Six aluminum water wavers used to create wavy hair, patented 6/15/26.

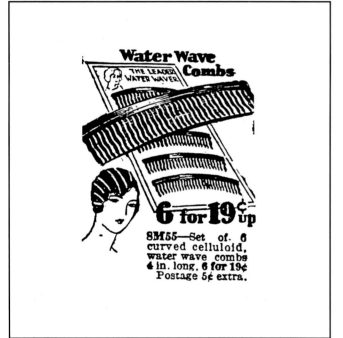

Water wave combs. / Aluminum (2 from a set of 10). *Courtesy of Rose Jamieson.* / Celluloid (2 from a set of 8).

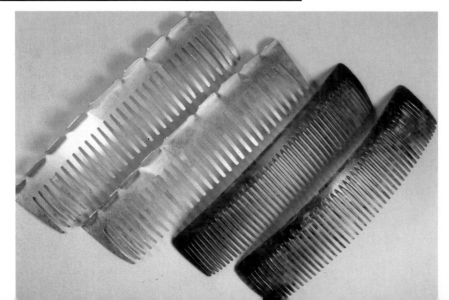

FINGER WAVES

"Finger waves" were another option. For extra holding power, a liberal dose of finger waving lotion was applied to wet hair. The hair just below the part was then combed to the left where it was held tightly with a finger of the opposite hand. The hair below this finger was then combed to the right, where it was held tightly by the next finger. After repeating this procedure several times, an undetectable hairnet (made of human hair) was placed over the hair to retain the wave until it was dry.

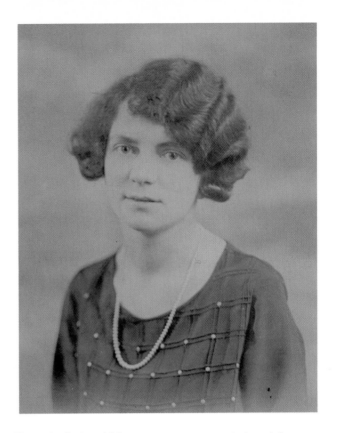

The author's Aunt Wilma in 1929, wearing a bob with finger waves. *Courtesy of Wilma Van Buskirk.*

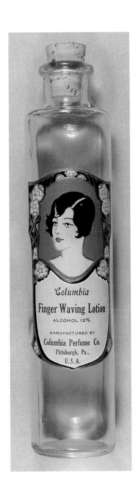

Bottle which contained finger waving lotion used to hold waves in place. *Courtesy of Rose Jamieson.*

Envelope containing hand-knotted human hair net sold by F.W. Wollworth Co., 1923. / Brown human hairnet. / Mitzi hairnet tin. *Courtesy of Rose Jamieson.*

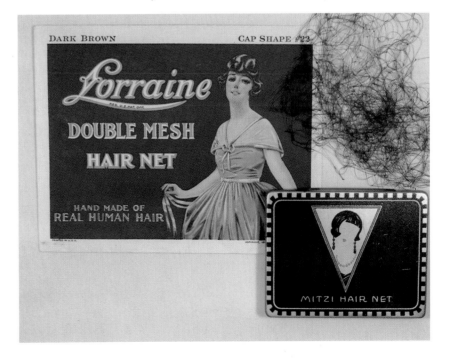

CHIGNON

Those who chose to retain their long hair wore it pulled back in deep glossy waves over the ears. It was then coiled into a chignon or knot at the nape of the neck. At first glance this style resembled a wavy bob.

Crimped wire hairpins called "bobby pins" were introduced for hair management. Fancy lace boudoir caps or boudoir *bandeaux* were worn to cover "rumpled" or "undressed" hair in the morning.

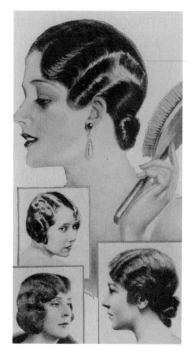

Top and right—chignon at the nape of the neck. / Left—two bobbed hair styles. *McCall's*, 1929.

Deep glossy waves ending in a chignon, spit curls at sides. *Courtesy of Rose Jamieson.*

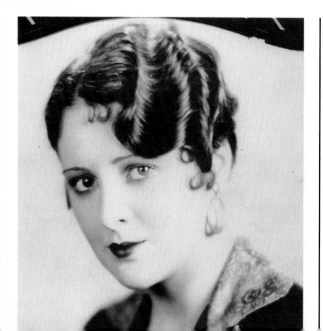

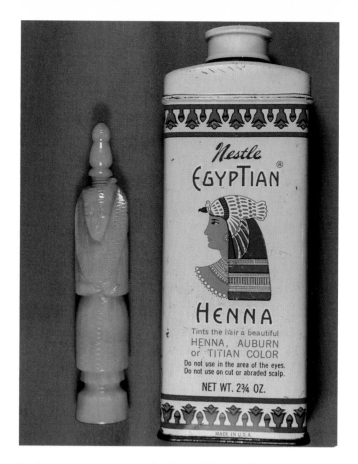

Bakelite perfume container in the form of Egyptian Pharaoh. / Advertising tin for Egyptian henna hair coloring. *Courtesy of Rose Jamieson.*

HATS

Hats were still *de rigueur* for day time. The variety of hats produced during the 20s ran the gamut from ultra feminine to severe and masculine.

EARLY STYLES

Hat styles from 1920-1923 were basically carry-overs from the preceding decade. They had deep loose-fitting crowns to accommodate women's long hair. They were wired and interlined with buckram and other stiffeners to retain their shape. Fabrics such as satin, velvet, rayon faille, taffeta, moiré, and crepe were often draped, pleated, or tucked over the crown. Common styles included tricorns, asymmetricals, toques, and turbans (introduced a decade earlier by designer Paul Poiret). *Tam-o'-shanters* were also offered in velveteen, wool, and silk plush. "Napped beaver" was commonly used for winter hats, while straw was used for summer.

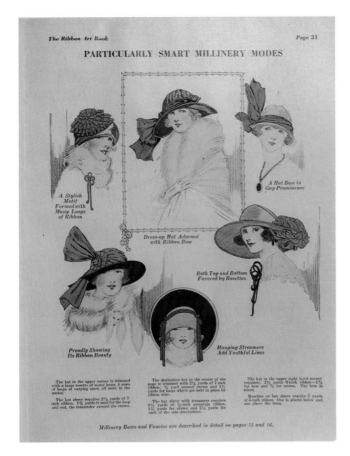

PARTICULARLY SMART MILLINERY MODES

A sampling of hats with unique ribbon treatment, published in the *Ribbon Art Book*, 1923.

Black velvet asymmetrical toque with feather trim, ostrich feather boa, c. 1919-1920. Label: Boyer, Allentown, Pennsylvania.

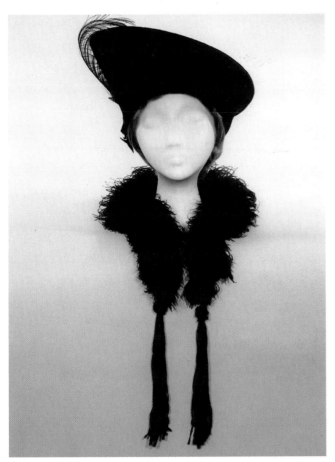

WIDE-BRIMMED HATS

A variety of hats with deep crowns and wide sloping brims were popular for afternoon activities, garden parties, teas, or visits to the beach. These hats were made of horsehair or pyroxaline (translucent imitation horsehair) and were often decorated with flowers.

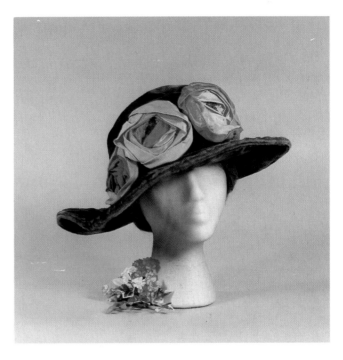

Brown velvet hat with asymmetrical brim and orange taffeta roses. Label: Reproduction of Mme. Georgette, Paris, by Tenné. *Courtesy of Jude Marsh (Kindred Spirits).*

Orange straw hat with deep crown, wide sloping brim, orange velvet band and flower.

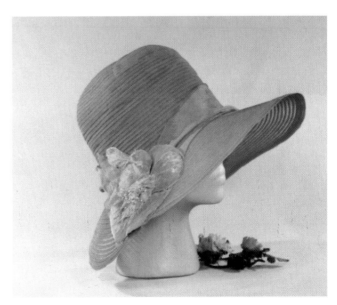

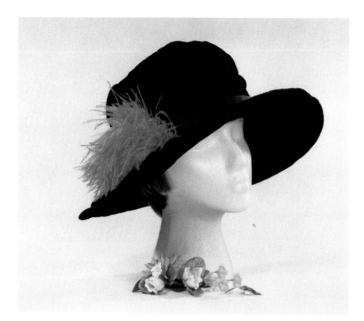

CLOCHE

Paris's leading milliner Caroline Reboux introduced the *cloche* style hat which became a trademark of the decade. *Cloche* in French means bell, which this hat resembles. Introduced circa 1923, it steadily grew in popularity until the end of the decade. Its deep snug-fitting crown and narrow brim covered the forehead (even the eyebrows) and concealed the hair to the nape of the neck. *Cloches* were made of satin, silk velvet, rayon faille, rayon horsehair, straw, felt, and solid or printed cotton. Hats at this time were usually lined with silk or rayon taffeta.

Black velvet hat, deep crown, wide oval sloping brim, grosgrain band, orange plume, c. early 1920s.

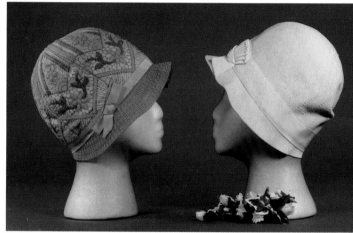

Beige quilted *cloche*, orange and green appliquéd designs, straw brim, grosgrain band. Label: Cedarbrook Models by Lyman. / White felt *cloche*, grosgrain band and ornament. Label: Katz Exclusive Millinery, New York, Chicago, and Paris. *Courtesy of Jude Marsh (Kindred Spirits).*

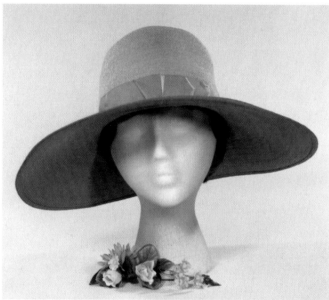

Orange straw hat, wide oval sloping brim, grosgrain band. *Courtesy of Ardath Peters Christine.*

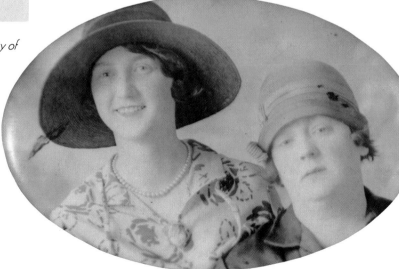

Author's mother-in-law Margaret and her mother pictured on celluloid purse mirror, 1926. *Courtesy of Margaret Laubner Stish.*

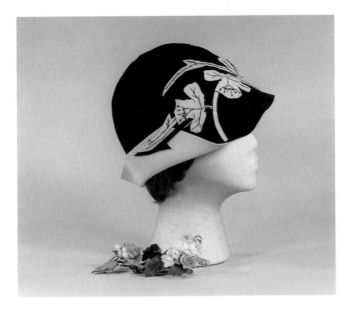

Brown felt *cloche* with beige felt appliquéd flowers. Label: The Lyman Hat. *Courtesy of Jude Marsh (Kindred Spirits).*

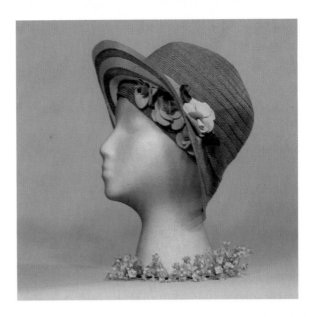

Lilac *cloche*, deep straw crown, asymmetrical brim made with alternating rows of straw and horsehair, decorated with pink gardenias.

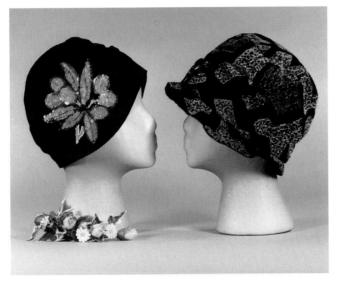

Black velvet *cloches*. / Orange sequined flower. / Abstract design of French knots in popular 20s colors. Label: New Ett models. *Courtesy of Jude Marsh (Kindred Spirits).*

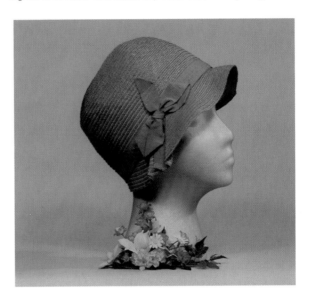

Brown straw *cloche* with matching grosgrain band and bow. Label: Gage Brothers & Co., Paris, New York, Chicago.

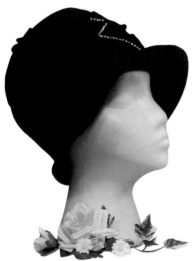

Soft black velvet *cloche*, rhinestone zigzag ornament. Label: Madelon, Paris and New York.

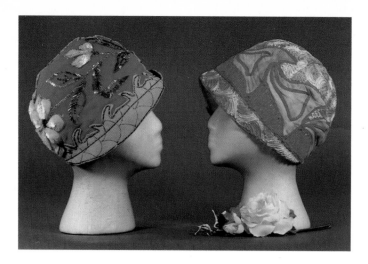

TURBANS

There were two types of turbans offered during the 1920s. The structured hat-style turban featured fabric which was draped horizontally over the stiffened crown and narrow brim. This type of hat was suggested for the mature woman. Reboux and her protégée Mme. Agnès designed soft wrapped turbans of knitted banding or crepe de chine.

Hot pink *cloches*. / Chiffon and felt with floral motif of pearlized sequins and bugle beads. / Felt with hot pink and cranberry soutache braid. *Courtesy of Jude Marsh (Kindred Spirits).*

GIGILO HAT

In 1925, Reboux designed the Gigolo hat which featured a tall crown with an irregular crease at the top. She is also noted for her asymmetrical "profile brims" which dipped lower on one side than the other. Reboux relied less on elaborate ornamentation than on unique shape, which she created through the use of tucks, pleats, creases, and asymmetrical cuts.

POKE BONNET

In 1927-28, there was a brief revival of the romantic "poke" style bonnet of the 1830s. This feminine style had a large up-turned brim and a liberal dose of artificial flowers.

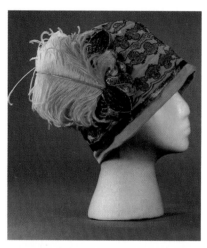

Orange *cloches*. / Velvet, gold metallic embroidery, orange plume. / Silk taffeta and straw, velvet flowers with green cord leaves. *Courtesy of Jude Marsh (Kindred Spirits).*

Cloche of brown and orange felt topped with brown felt *faux* bow. Label: The "Orb" Make, London.

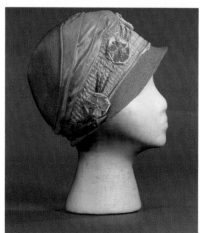

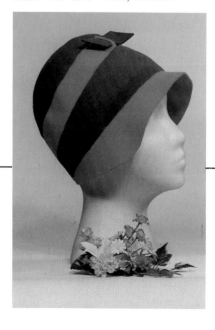

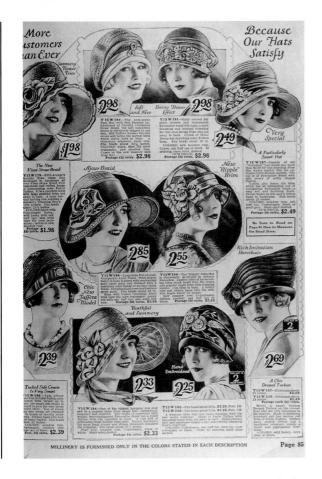

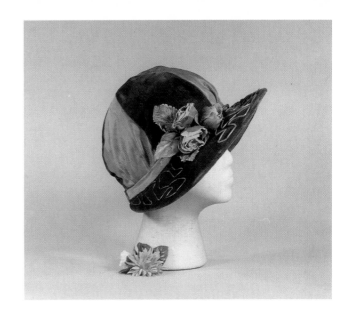

Brown velvet and copper faille poke-style bonnet, beige roses and leaves. Label: John Smith Co., Exclusive Millinery, Arcanum, Ohio. *Courtesy of Jude Marsh (Kindred Spirits).*

Hat styles featuring two tams, four poke bonnets, three *cloches*, and one turban (bottom right), National Cloak and Suit Co., 1927.

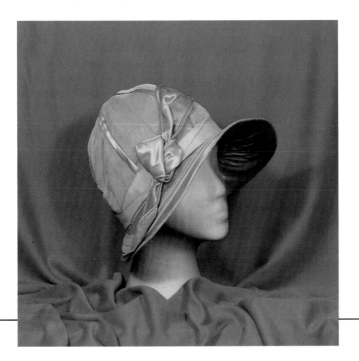

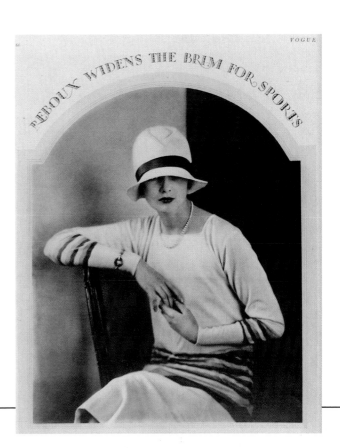

Rose beige velvet hat with deep crown and poke-style brim, trimmed in matching satin.

The felt gigolo hat, tall crown with irregular crease, designed by Caroline Reboux. *Vogue,* 2/27.

KNOCKABOUT HAT

The plain "knockabout" sport hat, with a rolled-back brim, was worn for leisure activities and horseback riding. The 1927 Sears, Roebuck and Co. catalog featured a knockabout hat which could be restyled by the owner to suit her own tastes.

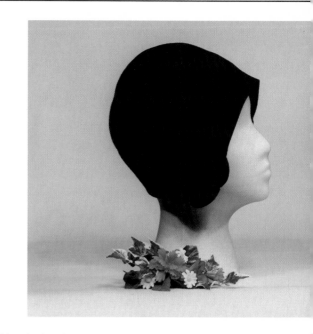

Molded felt *cloche*, deep crown, no brim, clover-shaped pieces of black felt attached over each ear, late 1920s. *Courtesy of Rose Jamieson.*

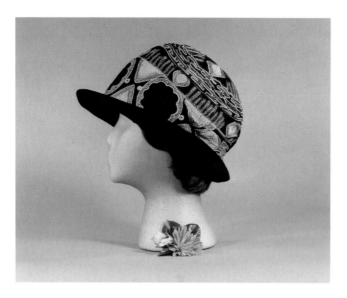

Black knockabout-style felt hat with rolled brim; orange, blue, and beige tambour embroidery. Label: Amour Hats, Paris and New York. *Courtesy of Jude Marsh (Kindred Spirits).*

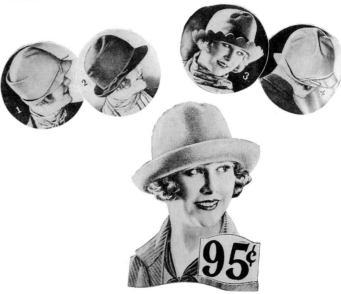

The "Knockabout" felt hat—(center) with regular roll brim, (1-4) show how a few stitches in the crown or a few snips of the brim could change this hat to suit a woman's own personality. National Cloak and Suit Co., 1927.

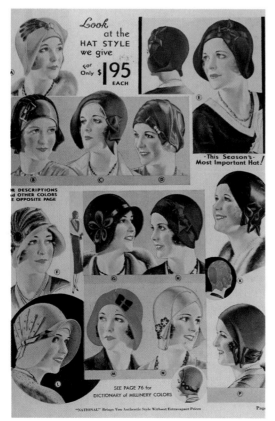

Cloche, forehead, and helmet-style hats. National Bellas Hess, 1930.

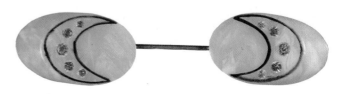

Art Deco-style mirror-image hat ornament made of bakelite with rhinestone ornamentation, late 20s.

94

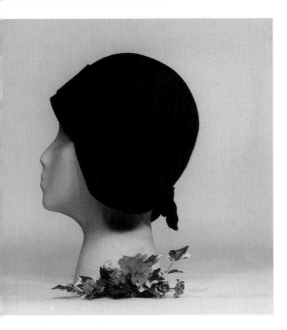

Forehead-style molded felt hat, black felt band over forehead and ears, grosgrain bow in center back, c. 1928-31. *Courtesy of Rose Jamieson.*

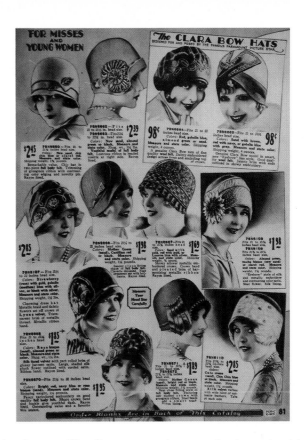

Hats featuring Clara Bow wearing the tam and turban styles. Note: special ear treatment on many hats. Sears, Roebuck and Co., 1928-29.

CUBIST DESIGNS

Avant-garde French milliner, Mme. Agnès, specialized in tailored sporty hats. She is remembered for her use of Cubist-style fabrics designed by renowned artists Piet Mondrian and Sonia Delaunay.

FINAL STAGES OF THE CLOCHE

The final, more severe stages of the *cloche* appeared in 1928. They were made of molded felt with no details beyond the silhouette of the head. The front portion of the brim was folded back, like a cuff, against the hat leaving the forehead visible once more; hence the name "forehead" hat. By 1930, the back portion of the brim was pushed down over the neck resembling a streamlined helmet.

TRIMMINGS

The most common trimmings used for hats of the 1920s were beading, feathers, braid, painted fabric appliqués, silk and chenille embroidery, silk, felt, or ribbon flowers, and grosgrain, satin, or velvet ribbons. Large flat flowers or ribbon wheels were often attached to the hat over each ear.

HAT ORNAMENTS

Art Deco-style hat ornaments became fashionable during the second half of the decade. They were usually composed of two decorative ornaments on either end of a short pointed metal shaft. When the shaft was inserted through a hat, only the decorative ends were visible creating the look of two separate pins. They were usually made of inexpensive materials such as zinc, celluloid, or bakelite and were decorated with rhinestones, marcasites, or dome-shaped cabochons.

NOTED MILLINERS

Other noted milliners of the 1920s included Maria Guy, Jane Blanchot, Louisa Bourbon, Suzanne Talbot, Le Monnier, Marie Alphonsine, Rose Descat, and Rose Valois.

EVENING BANDEAUX, TURBANS, NETS, AND CAPS

BANDEAU

When Irene Castle wore a *bandeau* or "headache band" in the mid-teens, millions of women began to tie all manner of things over their foreheads. Although this style originated in the teens, it is more closely associated with the first half of the 1920s. Glamorous evening *bandeaux* were embellished with rhinestones, sequins, beads, lace, embroidery, colored stones, and gold and silver braid. Caroline Reboux designed romantic feminine-style *bandeaux* decorated with artificial flowers.

Long delicate feathers from the egret called "*aigrettes*" (also spelled aigret) were often tucked into the *bandeau* at the center of the forehead. This was a carry-over from the sumptuous Oriental turbans introduced by Paul Poiret in the early teens.

Strands of beads were also worn over the forehead with beaded swags or fringe dangling over each ear.

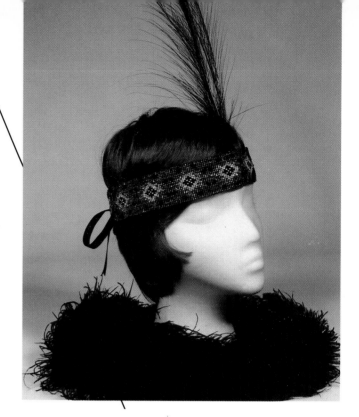

Bandeau decorated with rose, yellow, and black seed beads in the Argyle pattern, black aigrette. *Courtesy of Blanche Grabel.*

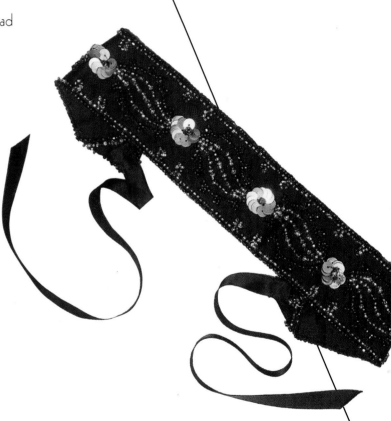

Handmade black grosgrain *bandeau* embellished with gold sequins and blue and gold seed beads.

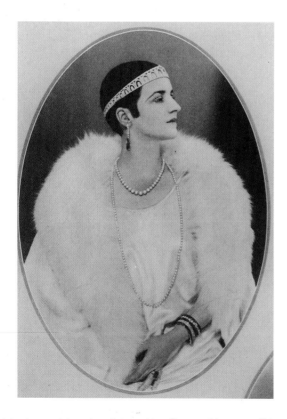

Flexible diamond *bandeau* designed by Cartier. Also note: Eton crop hair style, pendant earrings, white fox fur, long strand of pearls, and jeweled bangle bracelets. *Vogue*, 1925. *Courtesy of Richard Groman.*

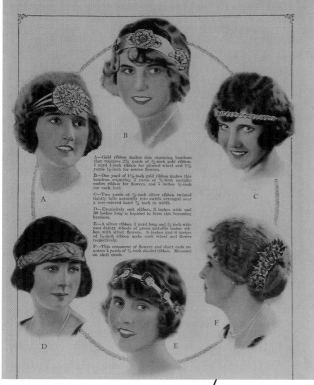

A BANDEAU CROWNS THE MODERN GIRL

A variety of handmade ribbon *bandeaux* from the pages of *The Ribbon Art Book*, 1923.

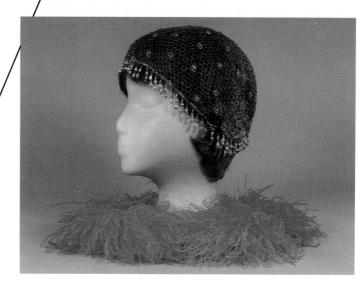

Silver hairnet with frosted pink and white seed bead rosettes and fringe. *Courtesy of Roberta Wickley (R & R Collectibles).*

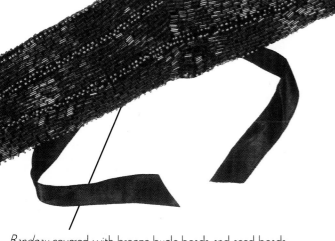

Bandeau covered with bronze bugle beads and seed beads.

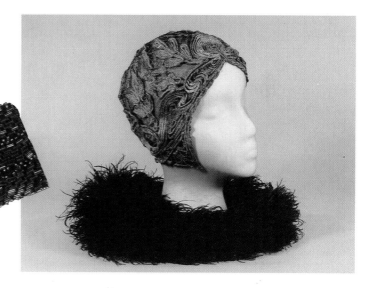

Evening cap of black net with gold braid and gold tambour embroidery. *Courtesy of Jude Marsh (Kindred Spirits).*

NETS, TURBANS, AND CAPS

Glamorous evening hairnets were decorated with sparkling beads and dangling beaded fringe. Elegant lamè turbans with an open crown were a specialty of Caroline Reboux.

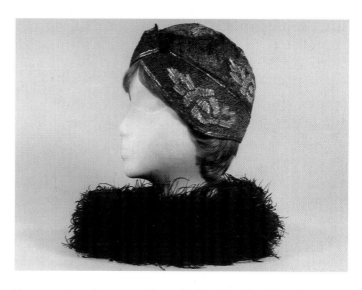

Evening turban of woven gold metallic threads and gold braided trim. *Courtesy of Jude Marsh (Kindred Spirits).*

BACK COMBS

Ornamental back combs and hair ornaments had adorned the most stylish heads from the early 19th century to the early 1920s. They were fastened into the chignon at an oblique angle, or were centered on the back of the head. They were enhanced with jewels or glittering rhinestones (primarily blue and green). The popularity of back combs began to wane in the early 20s, however, as more and more women succumbed to the call of the shears.

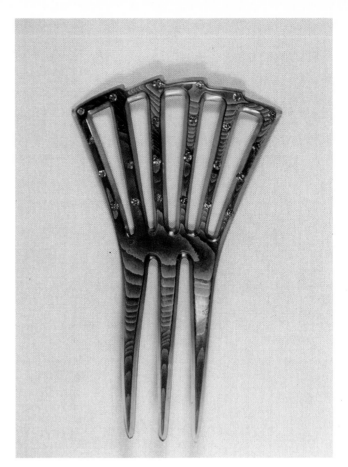

Fan-shaped marbleized celluloid back comb with blue glass stones, late teens to early twenties.

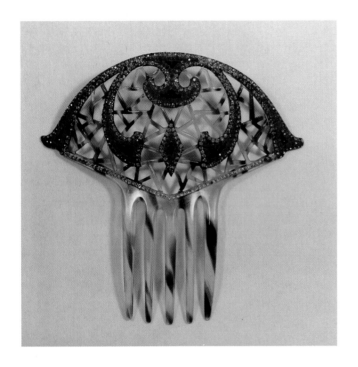

Celluloid (imitation tortoise shell) back comb studded with blue, green, and black glass stones, late teens to early twenties. *Courtesy of Margaretha J. Laubner.*

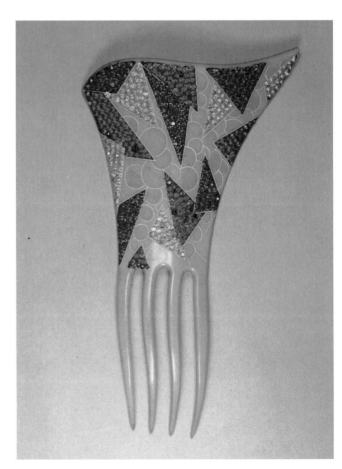

Art Deco-style back comb decorated with triangles of blue, green, and yellow glass stones. *Courtesy of Nancy Kintner.*

CHAPTER 9
HANDBAGS, VANITIES, AND COMPACTS

HANDBAGS

The independent woman of the twenties required a handbag in which to carry the daily necessities of life. Different types of bags were worn at different times of the day. Leather and cloth bags were used primarily for morning, while beaded and mesh bags were used with fancy afternoon and evening wear.

Bag frames were composed of a variety of materials to suit every budget. These materials included sterling, German silver (nickel silver), brass, steel, and gunmetal. Some frames were plated with silver, gold, nickel, rhodium, or chrome. The vast majority of handbag frames were die stamped with raised, indented, filigree, or openwork designs. They were further enhanced by the use of hand or machine engraving, enameling, and semi-precious or artificial stones.

Some popular handbag styles were produced for a decade or more, creating an overlapping of old and new styles. At times this makes handbags difficult to date.

LEATHER BAGS

Hand-tooled Leather

Hand-tooled leather bags were a product of the Arts and Crafts movement introduced in the late 19th century. This movement promoted handmade decorative arts as opposed to machine-made mass-produced products. Leather bags were usually made of English or Spanish steerhide with goatskin lacing. They were hand-tooled with graceful, free flowing Art Nouveau designs, which incorporated objects found in nature such as flowers and leaves with long swirling tendrils and various insects. The frames for hand-tooled bags were primarily made of gunmetal. As technology improved, machine embossing became an option for a more modestly priced line of handbags.

These popular leather bags continued to appear in fashion catalogs into the 1930s, long after the end of the Art Nouveau period and well into the Art Deco period. The patent date was often stamped on the inside of the frame.

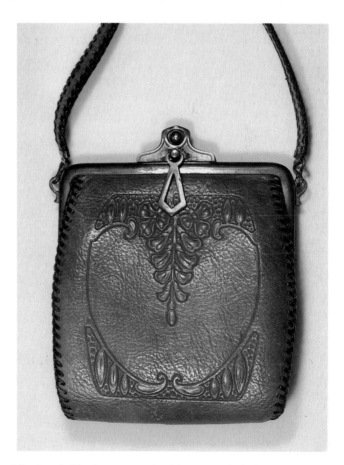

Hand-tooled leather purse - Art Nouveau-style fuchsia with swirling tendrils, gunmetal frame with opening tab, hand-laced edges and strap, equipped with coin purse and mirror. Marked: PAT 1/25/21 *Courtesy of Rose Jamieson.*

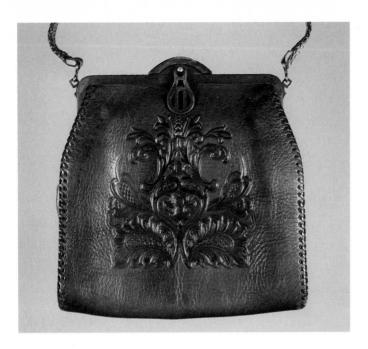

Leather bag with elaborate hand-tooled Art Nouveau leaf design, gunmetal frame with opening tab, olive suede lining. *Courtesy of Arlene Rabin Antiques.*

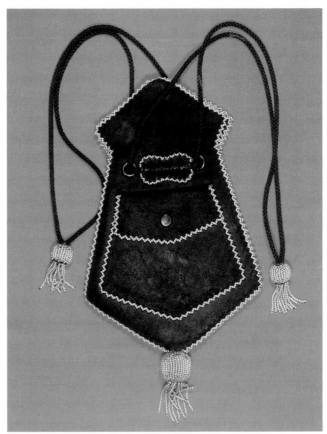

Black suede bag embellished with silver beads and beaded tassels, made in Long Island Veteran's Hospital by veteran of World War I, 1920. *Courtesy of Margaretha J. Laubner*

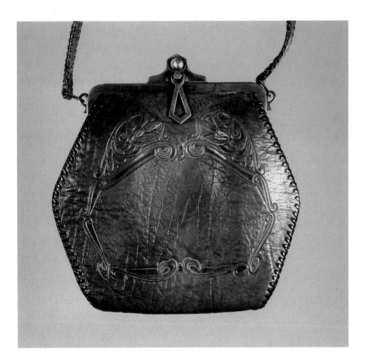

Hexagonal leather purse with hand-tooled Art Nouveau flower and scroll design, gunmetal frame with opening tab, hand-laced edges and strap, olive green suede lining. *Courtesy of Arlene Rabin Antiques.*

Pochette

The *pochette* or flat rectangular bag was introduced circa 1915 and reached its peak of popularity in the late 1920s and 1930s. These bags were either envelope style with a flap, or they contained a metal frame with a twisted-knob or fancy clasp. *Pochettes* contained either a short top strap, or a vertical strap on the reverse side of the bag. They were made of hand-tooled leather, leatherette, suede, tapestry, linen, patent leather, or felt. Smaller afternoon or evening *pochettes* were decorated with embroidery or sequins. These bags were carried by the strap, tucked under one arm (thus the name "underarm bag"), or clutched in the hand (thus the name "clutch bag"). Its sleek uncluttered lines made it ideal for modern Art Deco ornamentation.

During the second half of the decade there was widespread use of animal skins such as pigskin, lizard, alligator, crocodile, and snakeskin.

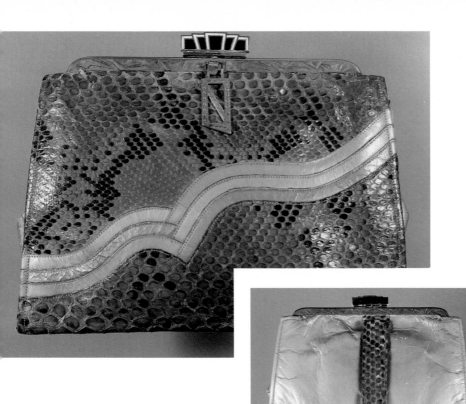

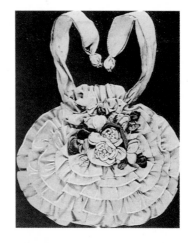

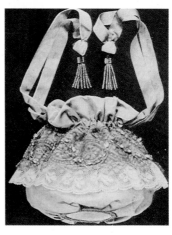

Front - snake-skin *pochette* with Art Deco clasp, frame, tab, and parallel leather appliqué. / Reverse - vertical strap handle typical of the late 1920s and 1930s.

Drawstring opera bags. / Blue taffeta ribbon, silk flowers. / Rose changeable taffeta, gold lace, French flower garland, and gold bullion tassels. Novelty Craft Magazine, 1921. *Courtesy of Suzanjoy M. Checksfield.*

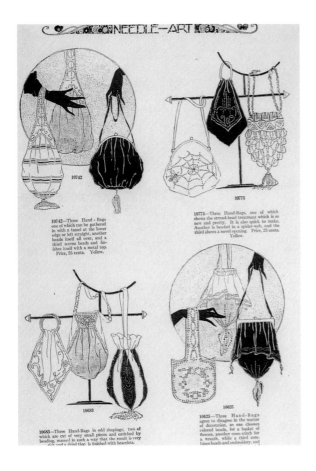

CLOTH BAGS

Handcraft magazines contained instructions for making "reticules" (pouch-style drawstring bags), bags which were gathered to metal frames, and *pochettes*. Kits could also be purchased containing all of the necessary materials to complete a bag at home. Needlepoint and tapestry bags played a limited role during the twenties.

A selection of drawstring, strap handle, ring handle, and framed cloth bags from the pages of *Needle Art* magazine, 1920.

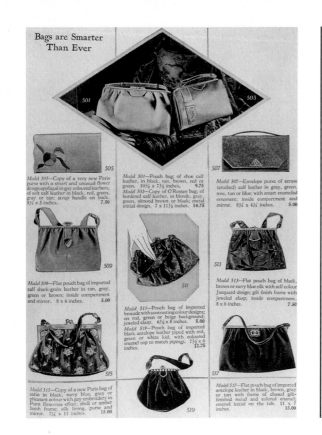

A sampling of cloth and leather bags in pouch and *pochette* styles. Franklin Simon, 1926. *Courtesy of the Kemerer Museum, gift of Barbara Stout.*

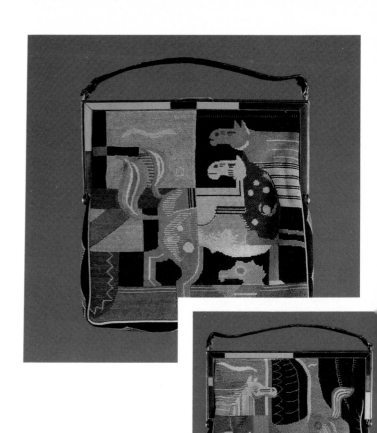

Fine petit point bag—Cubist-style horse illustrations on either side of bag, Art Deco-style enameled frame. Marked: Made in Austria. *Courtesy of Arlene Rabin Antiques.*

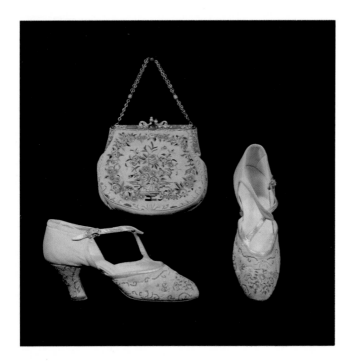

Petit point handbag, ornate frame with bezel-set glass *cabochons.* / Matching T-strap petit point shoes. *Courtesy of the Kemerer Museum, gift of Nina Mackall.*

BEADED BAGS

Glass Beads

Two sizes of glass beads were used for the embellishment of bags, namely *rocaille* (small seed beads), and slightly larger round or faceted beads. Both sizes were produced in a variety of styles including opaque, translucent, transparent, carnival glass (iridescent), opalescent, silver foil-lined, and cut steel.

Crocheted or knitted reticules were decorated with small beaded designs or were completely covered with beads or shaggy beaded fringe. The drawstring was laced through decorative holes, a tunnel in the bag, or through plastic rings or loops stitched to the top of the bag.

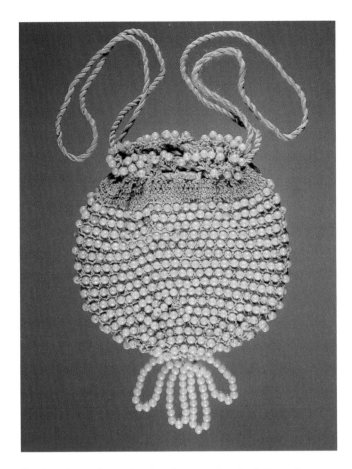

Crocheted reticule—white beads painted to look like iridescent orange carnival glass, c. early 1920s.

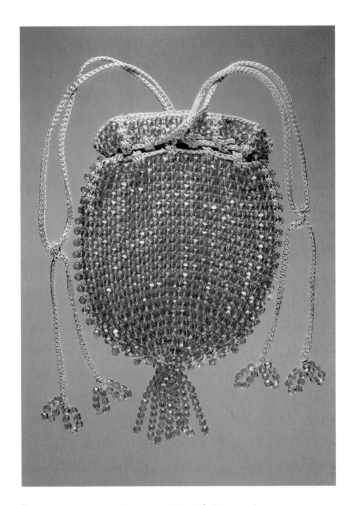

Crocheted reticule—Nile green glass beads, c. early 1920s.

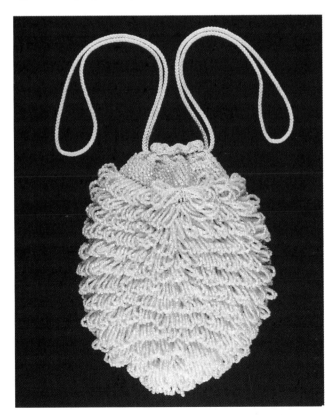

White crocheted reticule with rows of shaggy beaded loops. *Courtesy of Richard Groman.*

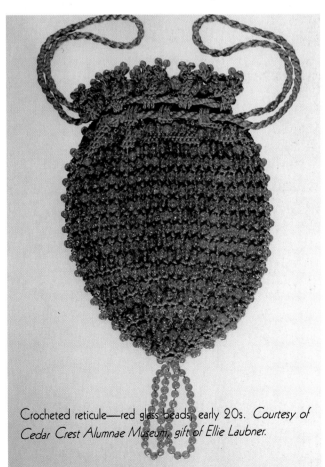

Crocheted reticule—red glass beads, early 20s. *Courtesy of Cedar Crest Alumnae Museum, gift of Ellie Laubner.*

Wrist strap bags had a 3/4 inch beaded handle which was an integral part of the knitted, crocheted, or fabric bag.

Beaded bags were also made with celluloid or metal frames from the materials mentioned earlier. Vertical beaded stripes were very popular for this type of bag, particularly those made of connecting diamonds.

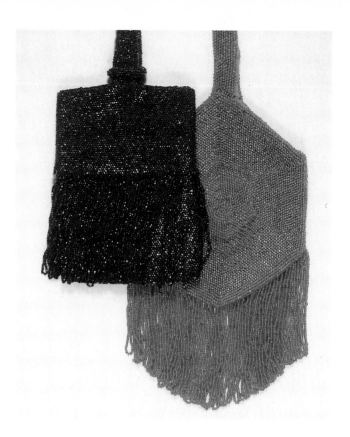

Two crocheted wrist strap bags with looped fringe, satin lining—Dark blue iridescent carnival glass beads, 1924. / Deep red glass and cut steel seed beads, 1924. *Courtesy of Margaretha J. Laubner.*

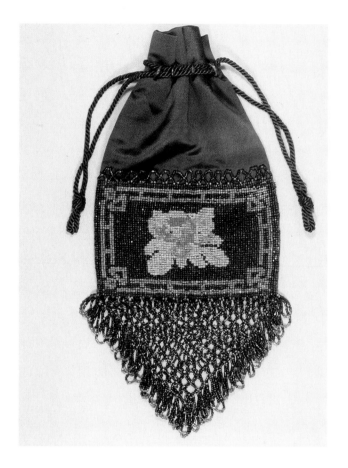

Navy satin reticule decorated with pink, green, gold, and blue iridescent carnival glass beads, ending with triangular beaded lattice work.

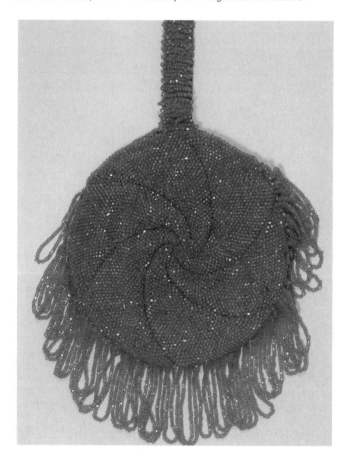

Handmade beaded bag covered with red seed beads in pin wheel design, beaded wrist strap, looped fringe. *Courtesy of Theresa Schouten.*

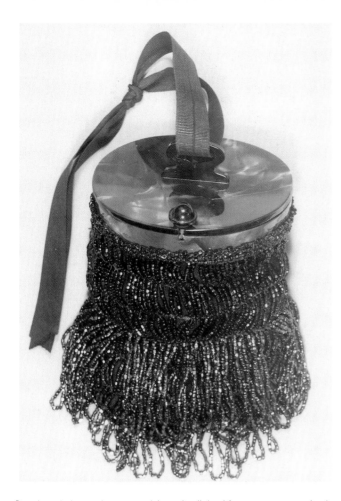

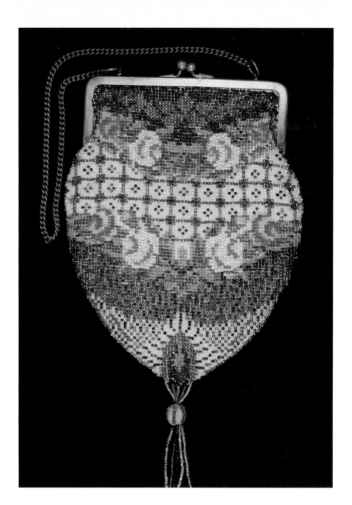

Pouch-style bag—brown marbleized celluloid frame, mirror attached to underside of hinged lid, covered with brown beaded fringe, grosgrain ribbon handle. Marked: PAT. APR.19,'21.

Beaded bag featuring pink roses, plain gilded brass frame. Marked: Germany.

Gable-style gilded filigree frame, bronze-colored carnival glass beads, long beaded-loop fringe, early 20s. *Courtesy of Nancy Blankowitsch.*

Fancy silver-plated frame with cutout floral motif, carnival glass beads arranged in stripes made of connecting diamonds. *Courtesy of Nancy Blankowitsch.*

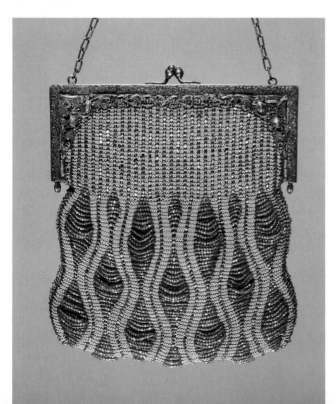

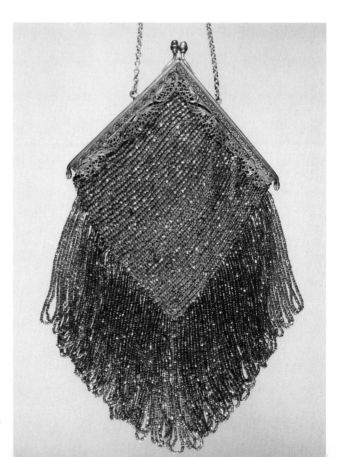

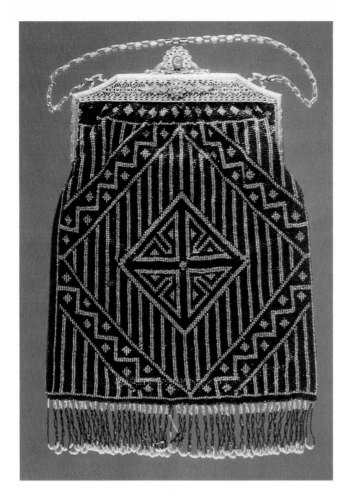

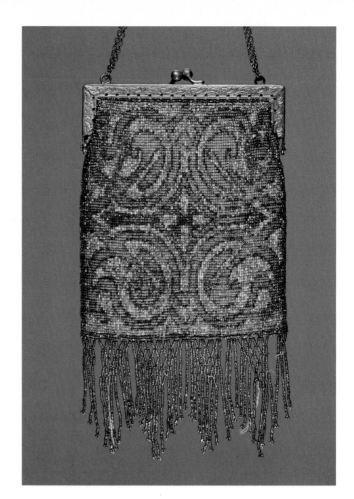

Marriage between gold-plated Edwardian openwork frame and Art Deco-style bead work design rendered in black and gold seed beads, c. 1925-30. *Courtesy of F. Paul Laubner.*

Gold-plated frame with knob clasp and double chain handle; brass, nickel, and cut steel beads; delicate lattice-style fringe. Marked: Made in France. *Courtesy of Nancy Blankowitsch.*

Cut Steel Beads

Silver-colored cut steel beads were still in use for a variety of bags. French bag designers in particular used cut steel beads which were chemically dyed to resemble gold or bronze. Brass and colorful Japanned nickel beads were often combined with steel beads, creating soft lustrous bags with subtle abstract designs.

Some beads which appear to be steel may actually be silvered jet. Since steel is the only metal which adheres to a magnet, it is an excellent means of testing for steel. Care should be taken not to wet steel beads as they do rust.

Those who wished to make their own beaded bags could refer to pattern booklets published by bead manufacturers or women's handcraft magazines. Kits containing purse silk, beads, transfer patterns, frames, and instructions were also available.

Woven beaded reticule with cut steel, brass, and jet beads; lattice-style fringe. *Courtesy of Roseann Ettinger (Remember When...).*

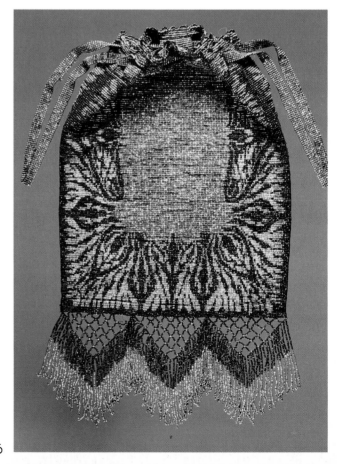

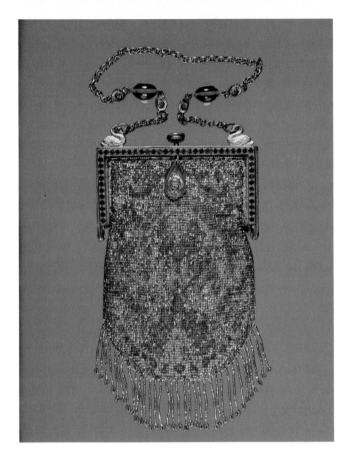

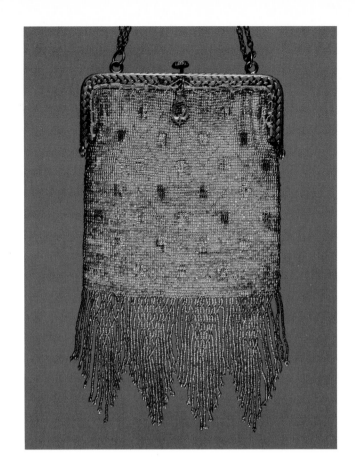

Gilded brass frame with swan terminals decorated with red rhinestones; push button clasp and decorative tab; cut steel, brass, and red Japanned seed beads; beaded fringe. *Courtesy of Richard Groman.*

Gilded brass frame with swan terminals decorated with green and red enameled squares and red glass *cabochons*; push button clasp and flower basket tab; enameled wide link chain handle; beautiful soft floral design made of brass, nickel, and colorful Japanned beads. *Courtesy of Nancy Blankowitsch.*

Gold-plated frame with raised braid design; push button clasp; double chain handle; brass, nickel, and polished steel beads; lattice-style fringe. Marked: Made in France. *Courtesy of Nancy Blankowitsch.*

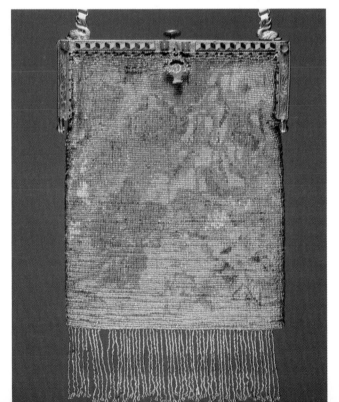

METAL MESH BAGS

Mesh bags came into popular use before the turn of the century. They were advertised in Sears, Roebuck and Co. catalogs as "a proper accessory for smart afternoon and evening wear." Due to their durable nature and wide spread popularity, these metal bags are now very easy to obtain.

The mesh portion of early mesh bags was fastened to the metal frame by the use of individual rings. By the 1920s, however, these pieces were joined by the use of an inconspicuous fine spiral wire.

There were three main types of mesh used in the production of handbags during the 1920s: "ring," "armor," and "beadlite" mesh.

107

Ring Mesh

Ring-mesh bags were made of thousands of small interlocking rings, resembling the chain mail worn by medieval knights. Originally, they were assembled by hand. However, in 1909, A.C. Pratt invented a mesh making machine which lead to the mass production of these bags in a fraction of the time, and at more affordable prices.

A man by the name of Dresden subsequently invented a machine which could manufacture minute rings used in the production of "fine" (or baby fine) mesh bags. As many as 100,000 of these fine rings were needed to produce one fine-mesh bag. Since these rings were so delicate, many bag manufacturers offered soldered fine ring-mesh bags at an additional charge. As incredible as it may seem, each tiny ring was individually soldered to provide a stronger more durable bag.

Many ring-mesh bags, of the late teens and early twenties, were long and unusually slender. They featured the "cathedral dome-shaped" frame which resembled a wishbone or house gable. Other bags were rectangular in shape with squared-off frames. Genuine or synthetic sapphire cabochons were often set into the knob clasps. Ring-mesh bags were fitted with a chain handle or a mesh wrist strap containing a moveable slide. The slide could be adjusted to secure the bag to the wrist.

"Sunset" mesh bags were introduced by Whiting & Davis, circa 1921-22. These bags featured fine gold, silver, and bronze-plated rings arranged in vertical stripes. Rectangular or elongated versions were available featuring fine chain fringe or a mesh tassel.

"Dresden" mesh bags (named after the inventor of the fine mesh making machine) were created by stenciling colored enamels onto the fine ring mesh. This procedure resulted in designs with a soft blurred appearance, similar to Chiné fabric.

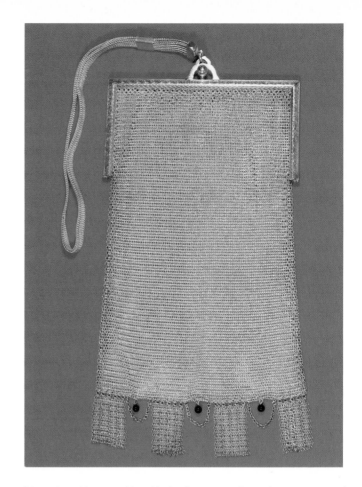

Silver-plated frame, soldered baby-fine ring mesh, mesh wrist strap with slide, ring-mesh fringe and swags. Hallmark: BB, sol'd (soldered) mesh, silver plate. *Courtesy of F. Paul Laubner*

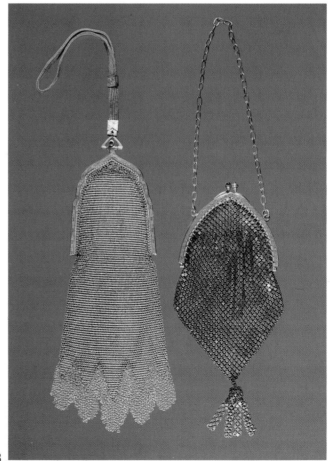

Two silver-plated bags with cathedral dome-shaped frames, simulated sapphires set in clasps. / Fine ring-mesh bag, mesh wrist strap with slide. Marked: Whiting & Davis. / Armor-mesh bag, fringed tassel. Late teens-early 20s. *Courtesy of Richard Groman.*

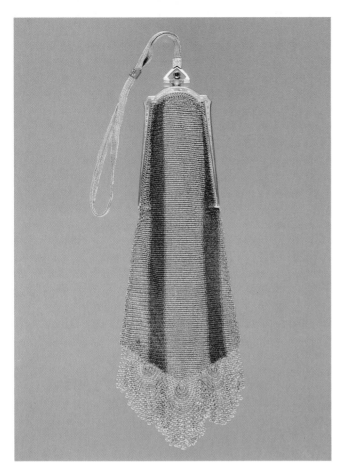

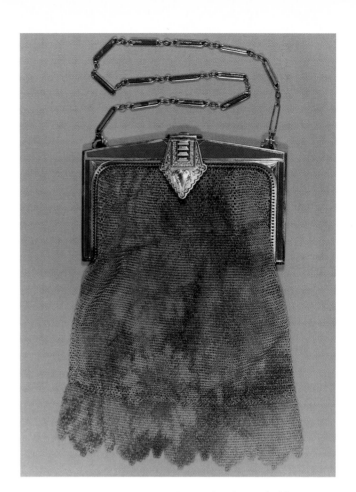

Sunset-mesh bag, gold-plated cathedral dome-shaped frame with blue *cabochon* set in clasp, stripes of silver, gold, and bronze-plated baby-fine ring mesh, decorative fringe, mesh wrist strap handle with slide. Marked: Whiting & Davis, PAT D, Soldered Mesh.

Dresden-mesh bag, gold-plated frame with step clasp, enameled rose and forget-me-not design, *baton* link chain handle. *Courtesy of Nancy Blankowitsch.*

Dresden baby-fine ring-mesh bag, chrome-plated enameled frame, enameled floral motif, *baton* link chain. *Courtesy of the Kemerer Museum, gift of Helen Harvey Jones.*

Two Dresden bags, enameled baby-fine mesh, gold-plated frames, enameled abstract designs. / First bag marked: soldered mesh, Whiting & Davis. *Courtesy of Richard Groman.*

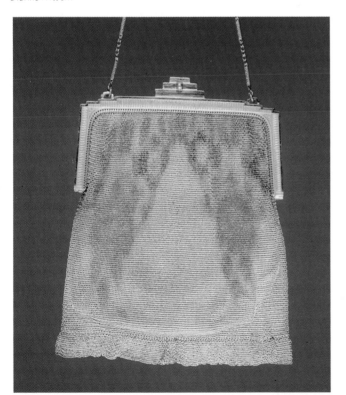

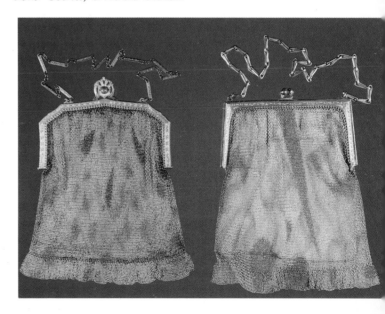

Armor Mesh

Armor mesh consisted of tiny flat metal links resembling multiplication signs (when used on the straight) or plus signs (when used on the bias). The four points of each link were bent and then hooked into adjacent rings on the reverse side of the bag. Armor-mesh bags were stenciled with colored enamels in geometric and stylized floral designs which were typical of the Art Deco period.

The *"Princess Mary"* bag, offered by Whiting & Davis in 1922, had an unusual frame which resembled the flap of an envelope. This bag was offered in ring, sunset, and armor mesh with Bacchus, Egyptian (zigzag), or fancy Venetian-style (rosette) fringe. It was named after Princess Mary, the sister of King George VI of England, who married Viscount Lascelles in 1922.

The *"gatetop"* purse was introduced in the 1880s. It consisted of a ring or armor-mesh pouch attached to a circular lattice-like expandable frame with a round hinged lid. To enter the bag the lid was lifted and the gatetop frame was expanded.

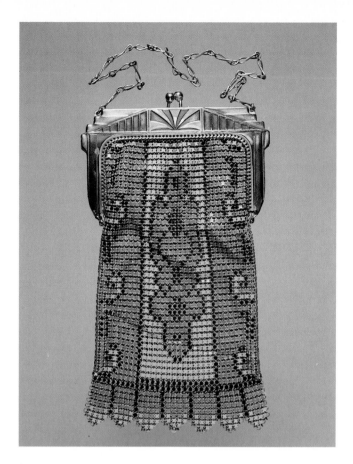

Armor-mesh bag enameled in Nile green and sunset orange, silver-plated Art Deco frame. Marked: Whiting & Davis. *Courtesy of Sally Meminger.*

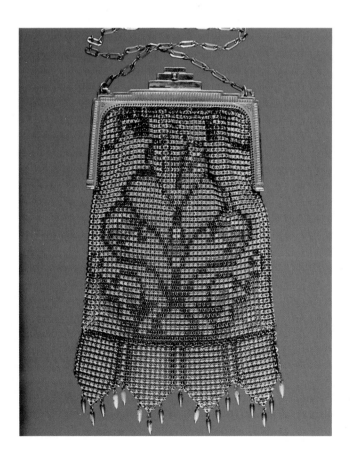

Enameled armor-mesh bag, gold-plated frame with step motif clasp. Marked: Whiting & Davis. *Courtesy of Richard Groman.*

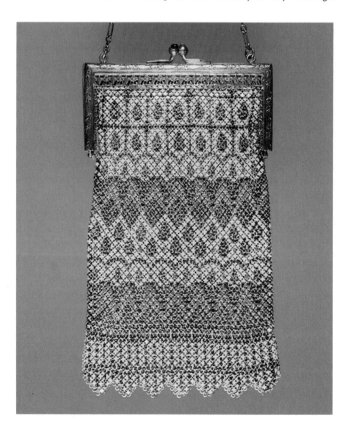

Armor-mesh bag enameled in Art Deco geometric design, nickel silver openwork frame, simulated sapphires set in knob clasp. Marked: Mandalian Mfg. Co. U.S.A.

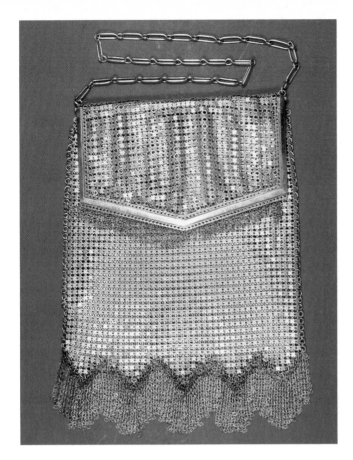

"Princess Mary" envelope-style frame with flap—silver-plated brass, armor-mesh, chain fringe, 1922. Marked: Whiting & Davis. *Courtesy of Inez Getty.*

Beadlite Mesh

Beadlite mesh, a variation of armor mesh, was introduced in the late 1920s. Each small link contained a raised dome-shaped center resembling a small bead.

MAJOR MESH BAG MANUFACTURERS

The *Whiting & Davis Company*, which originated in Plainville, Massachusetts, has been a leading manufacturer of mesh bags from 1892 to the present. This company is known for its ring, Dresden, and armor-mesh bags which often featured a zigzag hem end. Whiting & Davis is also known for its wide variety of unique mesh vanity bags.

Whiting & Davis bags were stamped with the company logo on the inside of the frame or they contained a tiny metal logo tag attached to the inside of the bag. Paper logo tags were also used, however, they were often discarded leaving some Whiting & Davis bags unidentified.

In 1994, the Whiting & Davis Company relocated to new modern facilities in Attleboro Falls, MA. These facilities include the Whiting & Davis factory, the company store, and a handbag museum. Among the museum's holdings is a pattern book containing many of the company's original designs.

The *Mandalian Manufacturing Company* was founded by Turkish emigrant Sahatiel Mandalian circa 1898. This company is best known for its armor-mesh bags which were enameled in wonderful rich color combinations. The most common motifs were stylized flowers, birds, and patterns resembling Oriental rugs (a reflection of Mandalian's Turkish ancestry). Many of these high quality bags contained ornate filigree or openwork frames which were often enameled or encrusted with glass or semi-precious stones.

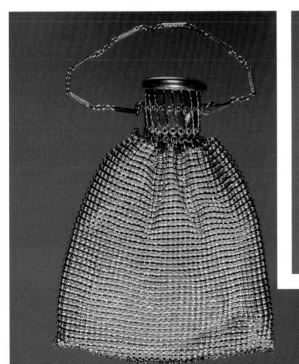

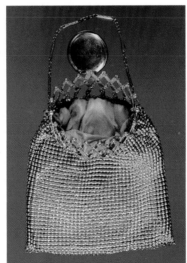

Closed - beadlite-mesh bag with expansion gatetop frame, *baton* link chain. Open - expanded gate, reveals gray silk lining, c. late 20s-30s.

111

The hem ends of Mandalian bags usually formed a large V or two inverted Vs. The hems were then decorated with fine chain fringe or enameled teardrop-shaped weights. These bags were stamped Mandalian Mfg. Co. on the inside of the frame. The Mandalian Company was acquired by Whiting & Davis in 1944.

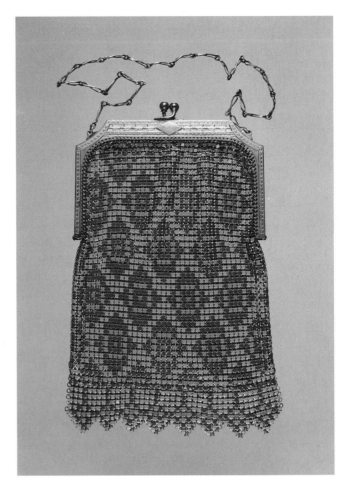

Armor-mesh bag enameled in diamond pattern, gold-plated frame. Marked: Whiting & Davis. *Courtesy of Sally Meminger.*

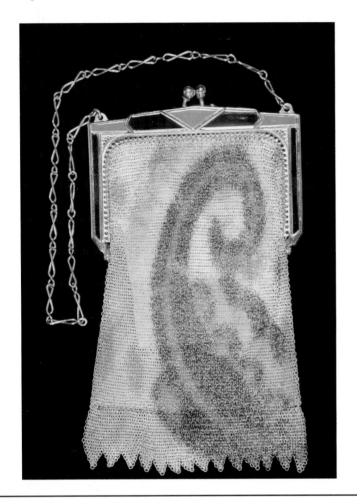

Dresden baby-fine ring-mesh bag, enameled Art Deco-style chrome-plated frame, enameled abstract design. Marked: Whiting & Davis.

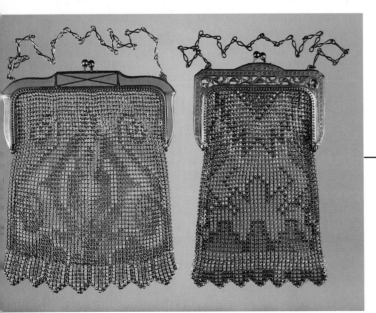

Enameled armor-mesh bags in typical 1920s colors. / Chrome-plated frame with blue enamel. / Silver-plated open-work frame. Both marked: Whiting & Davis. *Courtesy of Richard Groman.*

OTHER NOTED MESH BAG MANUFACTURERS

Other mesh bag makers of the 1920s include: the Bliss/Napier Company, Meriden, Connecticut; Henry Wiener and Son, New York; the John V. Farwell Company, Chicago; the Sanderson Manufacturing Company, Providence, Rhode Island; the Fort Dearborn Watch and Clock Company, Fort Dearborn, Michigan; the Automatic Meshbag Company, Providence, Rhode Island; Miller Brothers; and the R.& G. Company.

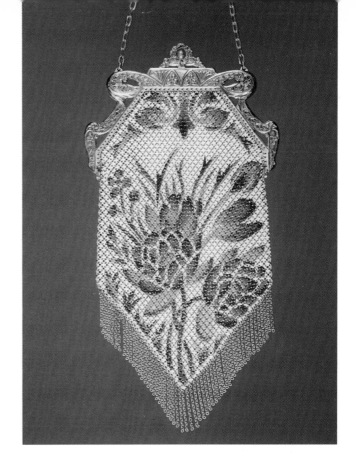

Armor-mesh bag, silver-plated Art Nouveau-style frame, stenciled floral design, V-shaped hem end with chain fringe. Marked: Mandalian. *Courtesy of Nancy Blankowitsch.*

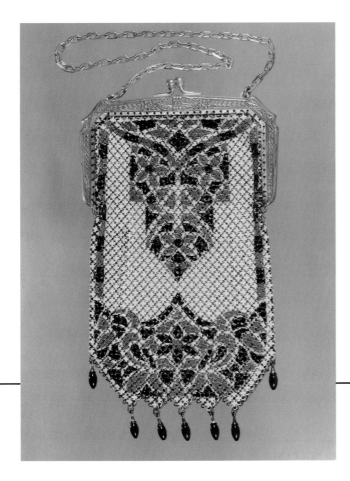

Armor-mesh bag enameled in stylized floral design, silver-plated frame, black enameled ornamental weights at bottom. Marked: Mandalian Mfg. Co. *Courtesy of Mary Alberger Pascoe.*

Enameled armor-mesh bag with raised floral design, ring-mesh fringe, and silver-plated cathedral dome-shaped frame. Marked: Mandalian Mfg. Co. *Courtesy of Theresa Schouten.*

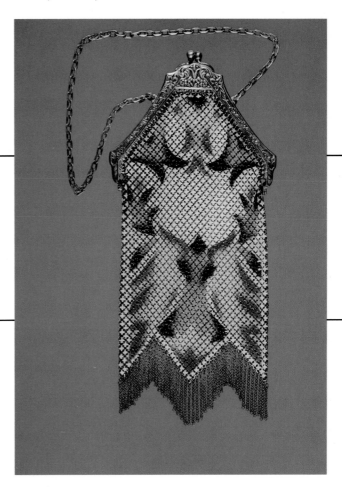

MESH VANITY BAGS

The shortage of young men created by the First World War made it difficult for many women to find a husband. Women's new-found independence and their efforts to appear more attractive to the opposite sex lead to the widespread use of makeup.

Powder and rouge were necessary to cover the shiny nose and provide a healthy glow. Bright red lipstick was needed to define the stylish "cupid's bow" lips. Eyes were highlighted with black eye shadow (made from Middle Eastern kohl), and eyebrows were plucked into pencil thin arches. The growing popularity of cosmetics created a need for vanity bags and cases in which to carry these all important items.

"For those moments which you simply couldn't face unless you were sure your nose was properly powdered," the Napier-Bliss Company of North Attleboro, Massachusetts, created the Du Barry vanity bag in 1921. This ring-mesh bag with a cathedral dome-shaped frame, featured a small powder compact which was attached to the clasp by a single braided-mesh chain. The compact contained pressed powder and a small mirror. The bag was carried by placing the compact in the palm of the hand and allowing the chain to slip between two of the fingers.

Du Barry soldered baby fine ring-mesh vanity bag, engraved cathedral dome-shaped frame, engraved powder compact attached with braided-mesh chain. Marked: Bliss, sterling. *Courtesy of Roseann Ettinger (Remember When....).*

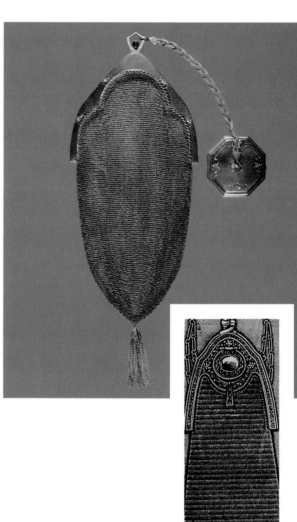

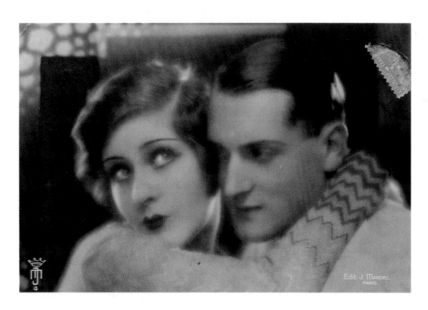

French postcard depicts flapper with pencil thin eyebrows, eye shadow, mascara, and painted cupid's bow lips.

Silver-plated Piccadilly ring-mesh vanity bag, cathedral dome-shap[ed] frame features round powder compartment with tiny pull tab. Se[ars] Roebuck and Co. 1923.

DEAUVILLE VANITY BAG

A similar example, called the Deauville vanity bag, was produced (circa 1922) by the Miller Brothers Company of New York. In this case the compact was attached to the mesh wrist-strap handle.

PICCADILLY VANITY BAG

The Piccadilly mesh vanity bag contained a small round powder compact built into its frame. A slight tug on the small metal tab released the spring loaded lid revealing a mirror, powder, and round powder puff. Piccadilly bags were produced in both ring and armor mesh.

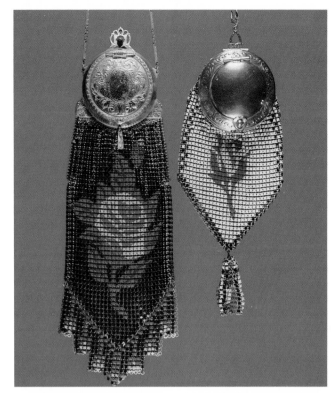

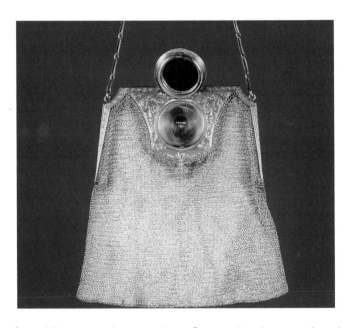

Piccadilly ring-mesh vanity bag. Frame - hand-engraved and monogrammed, round built-in powder compartment with small mirror, blue glass *cabochons* set in knob clasp. Marked: sterling, WB. *Courtesy of Arlene Rabin Antiques.*

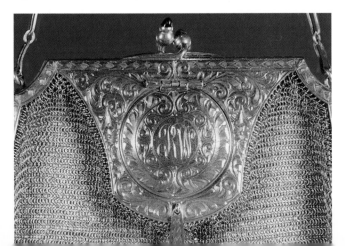

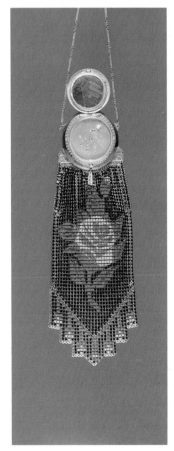

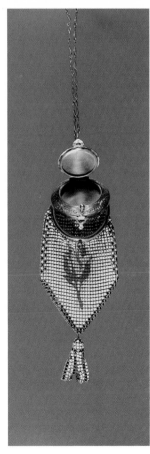

Two enameled armor-mesh Piccadilly vanity bags. Both have dual entry—one to the powder compartment, the other to interior of bag. / Gold plate over brass, entry to interior through top clasp. / Silver-plated frame. Both marked: Whiting & Davis. *Courtesy of Arlene Rabin Antiques.*

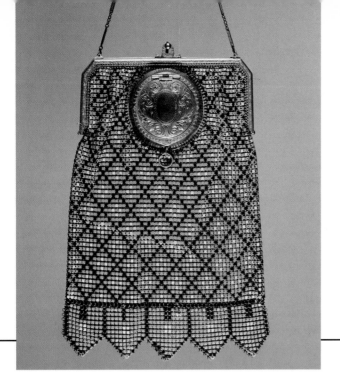

RECTANGULAR LID VANITY BAG

Whiting & Davis produced another line of ring and armor-mesh vanity bags with a variety of decorative rectangular lids. The gold or silver-plated lids were decorated with enameled floral and fruit motifs, filigree work and colored stones superimposed over multicolored armor mesh, or silhouettes of dancing nymphs or 18th century couples. (During the years 1920-1925 in particular, there was a revival of Rococo-style art, featuring 18th century figures with delicate floral and scroll accents.) The lids were cleverly designed to hold powder, rouge, a mirror, and a small comb or a money clip. The bottom of these bags was made of fine ring mesh (plain or enameled) or armor mesh enameled in multicolored geometric patterns.

Enameled armor-mesh vanity bag, gold-plated frame and attached compact which contains powder and mirror, *baton* link chain. Marked: Whiting & Davis. *Courtesy of Arlene Rabin Antiques.*

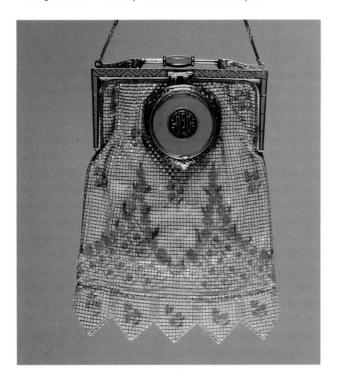

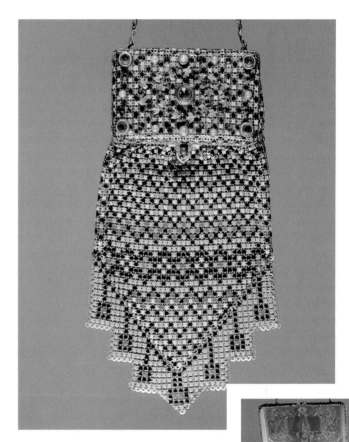

Rare chrome and enameled armor-mesh "Swing Compact Costume Bag," enameled frame with unique slide clasp, enameled compact with Oriental motif contains rouge, powder, and chrome-plated mirror, enameled *baton* link chain. Marked: Whiting & Davis. *Courtesy of Arlene Rabin Antiques.*

Enameled armor-mesh vanity bag. Exterior - armor-mesh, gold filigree, and *faux* jewels applied to rectangular lid. Interior - lid contains money clip, mirror, rouge, and powder with puffs. *Courtesy of Arlene Rabin Antiques.*

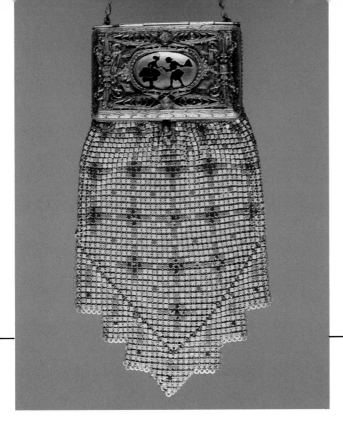

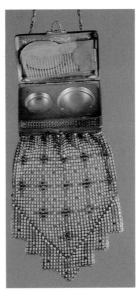

Enameled armor-mesh vanity bag. Exterior - gold-plated brass rectangular lid with applied filigree, green glass stones, and oval medallion enameled with 18th c. silhouettes. Interior - lid contains oval mirror, comb, rouge and powder wells. *Courtesy of Arlene Rabin Antiques.*

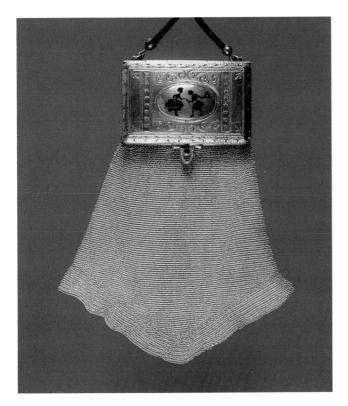

Silver-plated vanity bag. Exterior - rectangular lid with applied oval medallion containing enameled 18th c. silhouettes, cord handle with slide. Interior - lid contains oval mirror, comb, rouge and powder wells. Marked: Whiting & Davis, soldered mesh. *Courtesy of Arlene Rabin Antiques.*

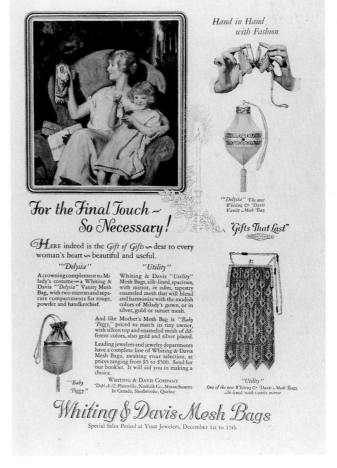

Advertisement for Whiting & Davis mesh bags. / Lantern-shaped "Delysia" bag, / "Baby Peggy" bag for little girls. / "Utility" enameled armor-mesh bag, 1924.

DELYSIA AND BABY PEGGY VANITY BAGS

The unique Delysia ring-mesh vanity bag by Whiting & Davis resembled a miniature Chinese lantern. This dual-access bag opened in the center with compartments in the upper and lower sections for powder, rouge, and a mirror. They could be purchased in sterling, silver plate, gold plate, and nickel silver. A similar bag for little girls was called the Baby Peggy. It consisted of a drawstring silk top with a gold or silver-plated ring-mesh bottom. These two bags were popular between 1922 and 1925.

POUCH STYLE VANITY BAG

A similar pouch-style mesh vanity bag was created by the R&G Co. The round sterling lid was decorated with hand-painted flowers over *gilloché* enameling. The bottom of the bag consisted of an enameled-mesh pouch terminated by a mesh tassel. The interior portion of the lid contained pressed rouge and powder compartments and a hinged mirror. The reverse side of the mirror was decorated with engine-turnings and a *cartouche* for monogramming.

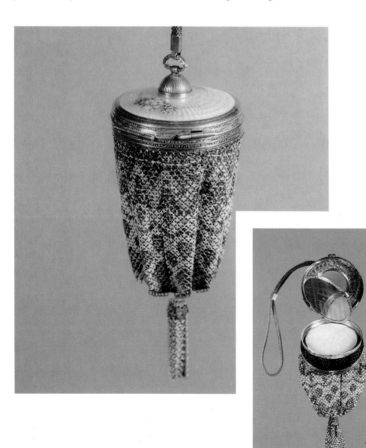

FORMS OF ORNAMENTATION

"Engine-turnings" were another form of decorative design used extensively during the 1920s. These machine engravings were incised into metal objects like jewelry, compacts, vanity bags and cases, and cigarette cases and lighters. Typical patterns were sun rays, basket weaves, concentric circles, kaleidoscopes, and rows of dots, circles, squares, diamonds, waves, and stripes which were applied over the entire object or used as decorative borders.

These engravings were often covered with translucent enamel which permitted the engraved grooves to remain visible. This process was called *guilloché* enameling. Delicate pink roses, blue for-got-me-nots, or baskets of flowers with blue ribbon bows were the dainty feminine designs most often hand painted over the *guilloché*. Finally an application of clear enamel was added for a protective coating.

Another enameling technique called *champlevé* was employed in the decoration of metal objects. In this case areas on the surface of an object are etched or routed out then filled in with enamel.

VANITY CASES

Vanity cases consisted of a metal, celluloid, or bakelite receptacle with a wrist strap, chain handle, or "tango" chain (a four-inch chain with an attached finger ring). Tango chains were often detachable so that the case could be carried in a purse or pocket by day (without the chain) or on its own by night (with the chain). Vanity cases were designed to hold powder, rouge, and a mirror. Larger cases were fitted with lipstick, coin holders (usually for a dime and a nickel), or a money clip. Many beautiful vanity cases were decorated with filigree and embellished with rhinestones, semiprecious cabochons, pearls, and marcasites.

Pouch-style enameled armor-mesh vanity bag. Exterior - sterling lid decorated with hand-painted flowers over *guilloché* sunray, pouch ends in mesh tassel. / Interior - lid contains rouge, hinged mirror (reverse side engine-turnings and monogram on *cartouche*), pressed powder. Marked: R&G Co. *Courtesy of Arlene Rabin Antiques.*

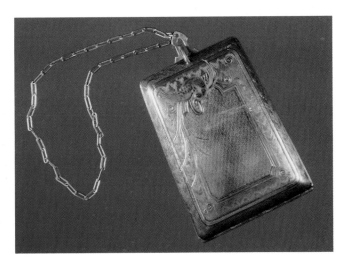

Silver-plated vanity case. Exterior - embossed bird motif with engine-turnings. Interior - mirror, powder well, and coin holders. *Courtesy of Sally Meminger.*

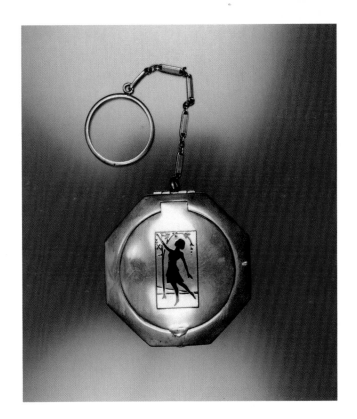

Octagonal double vanity case. Exterior - *champlevé* enameled flapper silhouette, *baton* link "tango" chain with finger ring. Dual entry - (top) rouge, (bottom) powder and mirror. Marked: International CW sterling, PAT. July 18-1922. 263/SL.

Silver-plated vanity case. Exterior - die-stamped border design; applied bas-relief floral medallion set with green glass, floral urn with marcasite, *baton* link carrying chain. Interior - powder, rouge, black kohl eye shadow tube, lipstick tube, and mirror. Marked: Marathon.

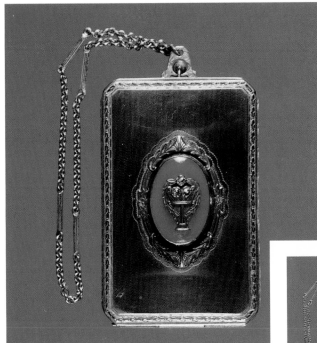

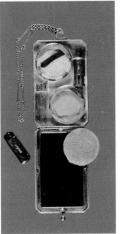

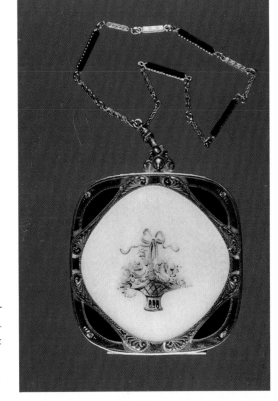

Chrome-plated filigree vanity case. Exterior - hand-painted flower basket over white *guilloché* enameling, enameled *baton* link carrying chain. Interior - powder, rouge, lipstick, and eye shadow stick (kohl). Marked: O.F.B. Co. *Courtesy of Roseann Ettinger (Remember When....).*

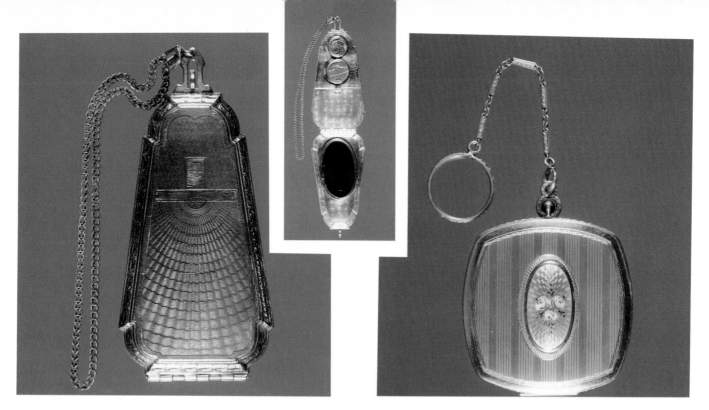

Nickel silver vanity case. Exterior - engine-turned Art Deco sunray motif, monogram *cartouche*. Interior - coin holders for dime and nickel, powder compartment with hinged door, and oval mirror. Marked: Evans, nickel silver. (Similar vanity case appeared in Sears, Roebuck and Co. catalog, 1927/28.)

Gold-plated vanity case. Exterior - brushed nickel-plated lid with engine-turned stripes, applied medallion with hand-painted flowers over *guilloché*, detachable *baton* link "tango" chain with finger ring. Interior - powder and rouge wells, mirror. Marked: FMCO (Finberg Manufacturing Co).

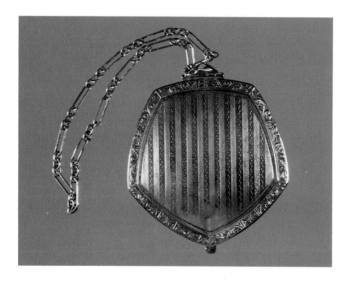

Silver-plated vanity case. Exterior - die-stamped border design, engine-turned stripes. Interior - powder, rouge, and mirror. Marked: Corinthian, Lodge No. 20, AF & AM, 1927. *Courtesy of Theresa Schouten.*

Black and white celluloid vanity case, black silk cord tassel. Dual entry - one side has powder and rouge wells with mirror; reverse side has empty space which could hold money or small handkerchief. (Similar vanities appeared in 1927-28 catalogs.)

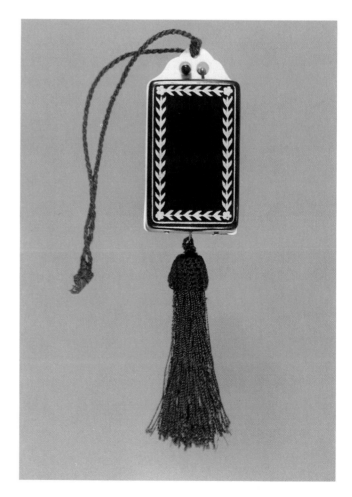

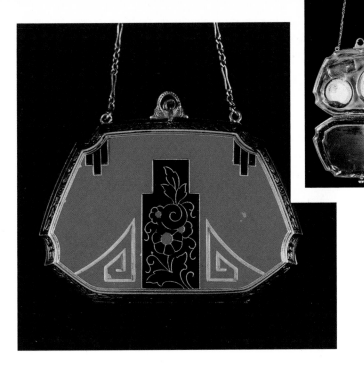

Silver-plated vanity case. Exterior - red and black Art Deco-style enameling, raised border design. Interior - lipstick, rouge, powder, and mirror. Evans, 1929. *Courtesy of Michele V. Weaber.*

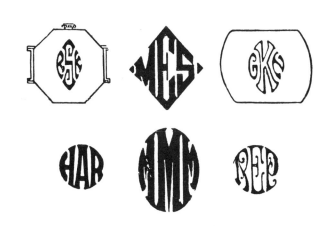

Necessaire. Exterior - *guilloché* enameled top, engraved sides, tassel (parted to show lower portion). Interior - dual entry - (top) powder, rouge, mirror; (bottom) celluloid slate, open compartment. / Lipstick tube attached by cord with filigree slide. Marked: F&B (Foster and Bailey) sterling. *Courtesy of Roseann Ettinger (Remember When...).*

NECESSAIRE

The *necessaire* was a small cylindrical-shaped vanity case ingeniously designed with compartments for some of the following items: makeup, cigarettes, handkerchief, comb, money, slate, pencil, or hairpins. These tiny wonders were made of a variety of materials including various metals, tortoise shell, celluloid, and colorful bakelite. They were decorated with enamel and precious or semi-precious stones. *Necessaires* were suspended on a silk wrist cord or carry chain, and usually ended in a long silk, beaded, or chain tassel which frequently concealed a tube of lipstick.

It is interesting to note that catalogs from the second half of the decade advertised metal objects decorated with sweet sentimental florals, side by side with hard edged Art Deco geometrics.

Monogramming was very popular during the 1920s. Smooth rectangular *cartouches*, designed for engraved initials, were frequently placed on metal objects such as: compacts, vanities, cigarette cases, lighters, belt buckles, and various types of jewelry.

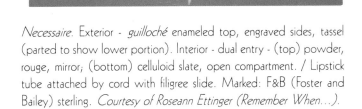

Many personal items of the period contained a small geometric-shaped *cartouche* for an engraved monogram. These are typical Art Deco monograms featuring letters which are confined to geometric-shaped boundaries.

COMPACTS

Small compacts were produced which held loose or pressed powder, a powder puff, and a small mirror. The loose powder compacts usually contained revolving sifters which regulated the flow of powder from the well beneath. Pressed powder compacts contained replaceable pressed-powder refills. Compacts were produced in a variety of geometric shapes including the circle, oval, square, rectangle, hexagon, octagon, and wedge.

MANUFACTURERS OF VANITY CASES AND COMPACTS

The manufacturers of these items were Evans, Elgin American, Foster and Bailey, the Ft. Dearborn Watch and Clock Company, the R & G Company, and the Finberg Manufacturing Company.

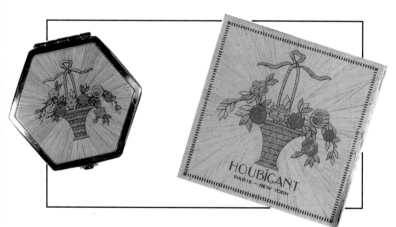

Small (1 1/2") gold-plated compact. Lid - stylized flower basket logo transfer covered with clear plastic protective coating. Interior - mirror, pressed powder, and puff. Marked: Houbigant. / Original box containing one refill.

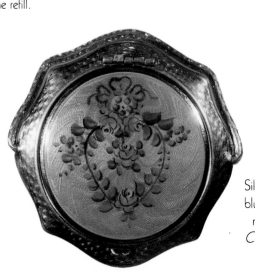

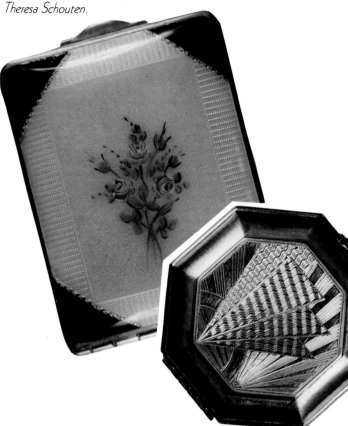

Silver-plated brass compact. Exterior - black enameled corners, *guilloché* enameling with hand-painted flowers. Interior - mirror, powder, and rouge. Marked: FMGO (Finberg Manufacturing Co.) *Courtesy of Theresa Schouten.*

Octagonal compact, silver-plate over brass. Exterior - engine-turned Art Deco motif. Interior - mirror and pressed powder with puff. *Courtesy of F. Paul Laubner*

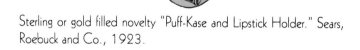

Sterling or gold filled novelty "Puff-Kase and Lipstick Holder." Sears, Roebuck and Co., 1923.

Sterling silver or gold filled powderette. Sears, Roebuck and Co., 1923.

Silver-plated brass compact. Lid - typical roses, for-get-me-nots, and blue ribbon bow hand painted over green *guilloché* enameling. Interior mirror and revolving sifter for loose powder. c. late 20s-early 30s. *Courtesy of Margaretha J. Laubner.*

CHAPTER 10
FOOTWEAR

During the first decade of the twentieth century, women's floor-length skirts stifled most interest in shoes because they were seldom seen. By the early teens, however, shoes began to peek out of the slits in hobble skirts. The entire shoe (or boot) became visible during World War I when, for practical reasons, skirt lengths rose above the ankle. Shoe manufacturers realized the potential that this newly visible accessory provided and began to produce more innovative designs.

With the eight-hour workday, paid vacations, and the invention of many modern time-saving appliances, liberated women of the 1920s had more time to devote to active and spectator sports. Shoe designers responded by introducing many of the classic sport shoe styles which are still worn today. The "spectator," "gillie oxford," "saddle shoe," "kiltie oxford," and "huarache" were all sport shoe styles worn during the 1920s.

Shoe styles were slowly evolving from the pointed toes and graceful curved "Louis" heels (named after Louis XV) of the early 1920s, to more rounded toes and either the "spike" or the thick "Cuban" heels of the late 1920s and 1930s.

EARLY YEARS

The John Wanamaker's catalog for 1921-22 still offered several pairs of high-laced walking boots which were on the verge of extinction. Also on the endangered species list were women's felt gaiters (spats).

Austere oxfords, walking boots with pointed toes and military heels, pointed-toe strap shoes with Louis heels. John Wanamaker catalog, 1921-22. *Courtesy of Suzanjoy M. Checksfield.*

OXFORDS

Laced oxfords with pointed toes and two-inch Louis heels (a carry-over from the teens) were still available. Sport oxfords were made with broad 1 3/4 inch "military" heels or low one-inch "walking" heels. (The heel measurement is taken from the front or "breast" of the heel.) Rubber soles and heels were introduced during World War I and were steadily gaining favor.

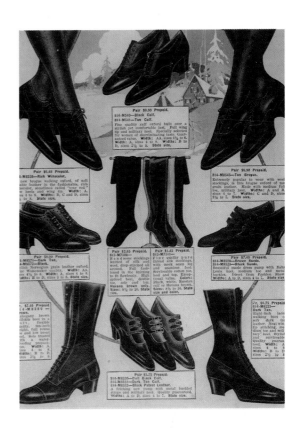

The 1920 Sears, Roebuck and Co. catalog advertised a brogue oxford with a military heel, trimmed along the edges and the wing-tips with broguings (small perforations).

STRAP SHOES

For dressy afternoon and evening wear, the buttoned one-strap shoe (called the "bar" shoe in the U.K.) with the French Louis heel was a popular carry-over from the teens. Variations of this style were the "two-strap," "three-strap," "cross-strap," and "T-strap" models. Straps on women's shoes had an important function during the 1920s, as they prevented shoes from sailing across the dance floor during the high-flying kicks of the "Charleston."

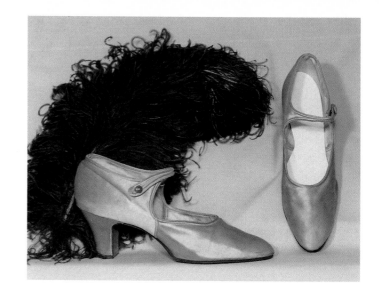

Peach satin evening pumps with buttoned straps, Cuban heels. c. 1925-30.

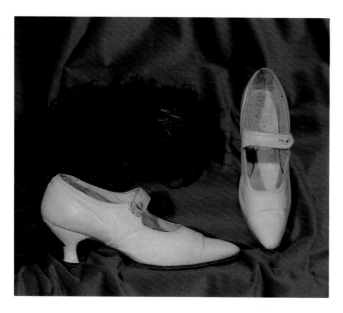

White kid buttoned strap shoes, pointed toes, curved Louis heel, c. late teens-early 1920s. *Courtesy of Betsey Pacini.*

Black kid cross-strap shoes, pointed toes, curved Louis heels, and black beading over vamp, c. late teens-early 20s.

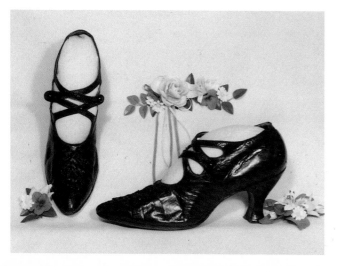

PUMPS

The plain pump ("court" shoe in the U.K.) remained popular for afternoon and evening wear.

The "colonial" pump, also a carry-over from the teens, had a large square or pointed tongue which extended over the instep (similar to those worn by English Pilgrims). The tongue was often decorated with a large rectangular buckle or ornament.

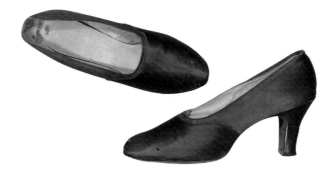

Pumps worn by a mother-of-the-bride, spike heel, 1929. *Courtesy of Pauline Weber.*

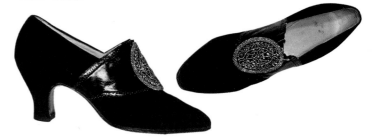

Black suede evening shoes, black patent leather saddle, cut steel ornament, Cuban heel. Marked: Saks and Company, New York. c. mid-1920s.

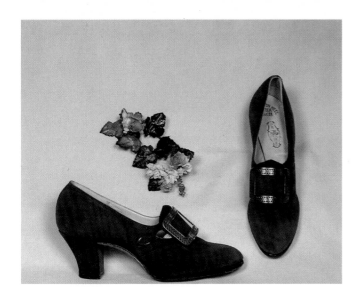

Adaptation of colonial pump—brown suede with gold-plated buckles and Cuban heels, c. late 20s-30s. Marked: Sautter's, Utica, N.Y.

THEO

The 1920 Sears, Roebuck and Co. catalog also featured the Theo, a tongueless shoe with one pair of eyelets on the instep strap. A ribbon was threaded through the eyelets, then tied in a bow. These shoes were sometimes called "Charleston slippers."

Shoes, at this time, were offered in a limited range of earth tones including brown, tan, or fawn for sport; and black, gray, or white for dressy afternoon and evening wear. Kid, buckskin, satin, or patent leather were the primary materials used in making shoes at this time.

SHOE ORNAMENTS AND BUTTON COVERS

Evening shoes were made of gold, silver, copper, and bronze kid, as well as vivid metallic brocades and velvets. Large cut steel, brass, and rhinestone-studded ornaments appeared over the insteps of evening shoes. Pairs of small metal shoe button covers were created to slip over shoe buttons and thereby give the ordinary one-strap shoe a little pizzazz. Many of the shoe button covers pictured in this book were patented in 1922. Others are decidedly Art Deco, which dates them in the second half of the decade.

Art Deco T-strap evening shoes of silver and gold kid, Spanish heels. c. 1925-35. Marked: Daniel Green.

MIDDLE YEARS

T-STRAP

Evening shoes of the mid-twenties became more glamorous and sophisticated. The T-strap grew in popularity and was worn for day or evening. The narrow 1/4 inch straps were fastened with buttons or small decorative metal buckles. The Louis heel was replaced by the two-inch "spike" or "Spanish" heel which was named for the Latin American dances which were popular at the time.

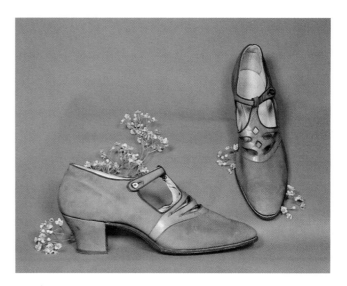

Gray suede T-strap shoes, tan cutout leather insteps, military heels. Worn with gray hose as wedding shoes in 1924. *Courtesy of Cedar Crest Alumnae Museum, gift of Betty Guman.*

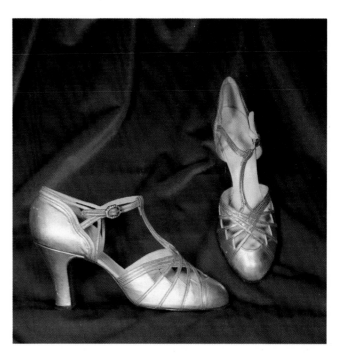

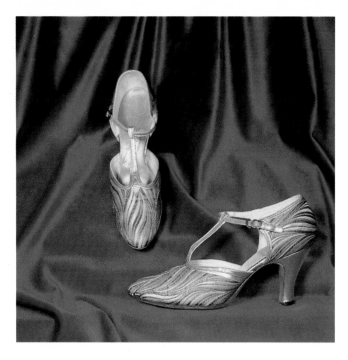

T-strap evening shoes, brocade with gold and silver kid, Spanish heels, c. mid-1920s. Marked: Frank Brothers, New York.

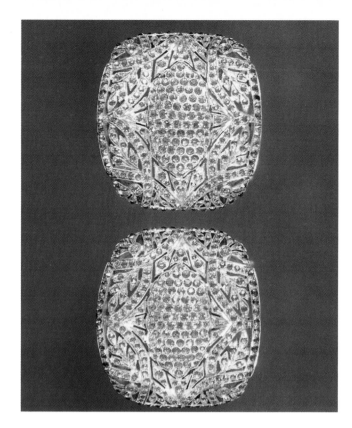

Chrome-plated shoe ornaments with *pavé* set rhinestones. Marked: Lord & Taylor.

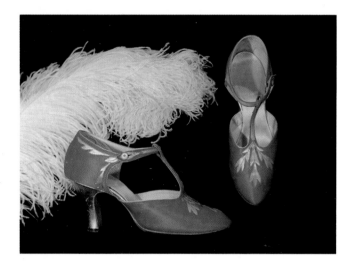

T-strap evening shoes, red satin, gold kid Spanish heels and appliqué work, c. mid-1920s. *Courtesy of Betsey Pacini.*

Shoe button covers. / Cut steel. Marked: France. / Pavé set rhinestones on base metal. Reverse side reveals small bracket. Marked: PAT.PEND. / One brass Art Deco cover (mate is missing). [Directions—Thread the instep strap through the bracket. Button the button. Push the button shank into the notch in the bracket.] *Courtesy of Mary Anne Faust.*

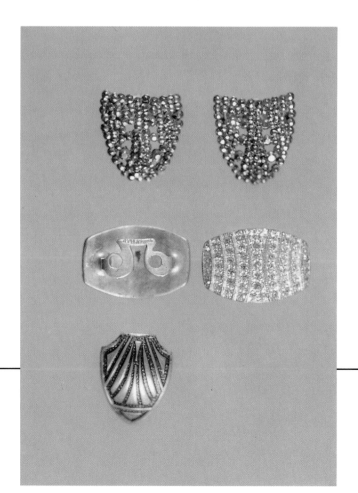

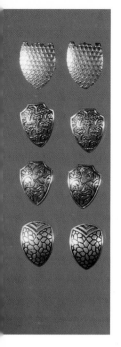
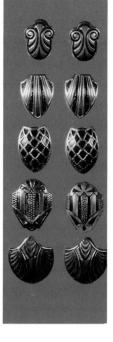
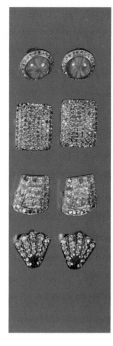

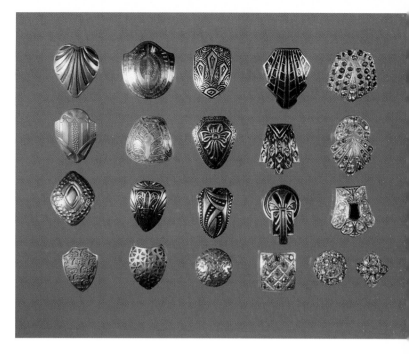

Pairs of shoe button covers decorated with enamel, rhinestones, and imitation star sapphire. Center row shows Art Deco influence. Many marked: Reyco, 1922. *Courtesy of Sally Meminger.*

Single shoe button covers (mates missing), brass and silver plate with enamel, base metal with rhinestones. Top two in second row have *guilloché* enameling. Many show strong Art Deco influence. *Courtesy of Sally Meminger.*

ANIMAL SKINS

There was growing interest in the use of pigskin, lizard, alligator, crocodile, snakeskin, and for the more modest budget, simulated reptile. Shoe manufacturers began to experiment with various textures, often combining two contrasting materials in the same shoe. One material served as the base for the shoe, while the other was applied as a trim, an appliqué, or an underlay visible through decorative cutouts. Typical combinations of materials were kid on satin, lizard on patent, kid on suede, reptile on kid, kid on brocade, and patent on suede.

KILTIE OXFORDS

The Scottish kiltie oxford featured a large fold-over fringed tongue under which the laces were tied. Some kilties were decorated along the edges with broguings.

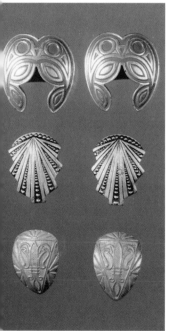
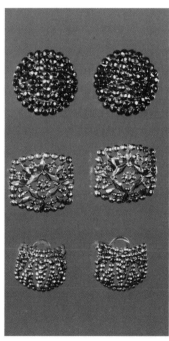

Shoe button covers. / Three pairs Art Deco-style of brass and enamel. / Three pairs of cut steel. / Several marked: France. *Courtesy of Sally Meminger.*

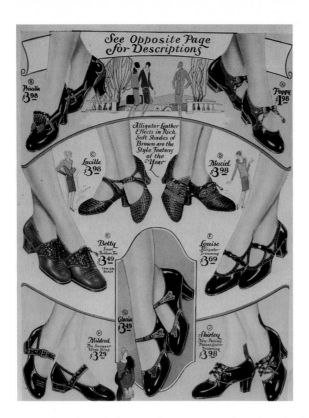

Good examples of rounded toes and extensive use of reptile and snake-skin during the mid-late 1920s. The Peggy (top right) is an adaptation of the Theo style. M.W. Savage C., 1927-28.

GILLIE

On his visit to the United States, the Prince of Wales (later the Duke of Windsor) introduced the gillie oxford, a Scottish dancing shoe originally worn with a kilt. It was also called the "Prince of Wales" shoe. This tongueless shoe had round laces which were threaded through leather loops, rather than through eyelets.

SADDLE SHOE

The 1926 Franklin Simon & Co. catalog offered a white buckskin tennis oxford with a saddle of tan or black alligator. This classic two-toned shoe was later named the saddle shoe.

In addition to the colors already mentioned, shoe designers added green, flesh, cream, champagne, cherry red, and deep purple; often combining two colors in the same shoe.

> (0) Kiltie-tongue oxford, low rubber heel. (1) Gillie oxford, military heel. (2) Two-tone oxford (saddle). (3) Oxford, Cuban heel (old lady shoe). (4) One strap, Deco buckle and cutouts, Cuban heel. (5) One strap, Spanish heel. (6) T-strap, Spanish heel. (7) "Modish" oxford, Cuban heel. Wanamaker's, 1929.

LATER YEARS

Shoes of the late twenties appeared wider and heavier than earlier models. They had medium round toes with either the spike, the military, or the new stout two-inch "Cuban" heels. Shoes became extremely ornate with broguings, buckles, and bows.

OXFORDS WITH CUBAN HEELS

Oxfords with tasseled laces were now made with a stout Cuban or military heel. Ederly people tend to resist change, clinging to the old familiar styles of the past. As I was growing up in the 1940s and 1950s, I noticed older women wearing laced oxford shoes with stout Cuban heels. At the time, we thought of them as "old lady" shoes. However, it is interesting to note that these same shoes were considered quite fashionable during the late 1920s and 1930s, when these women were young and style conscious.

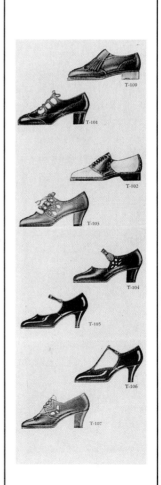

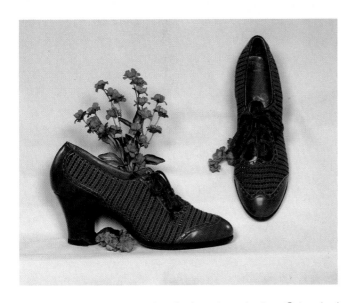

Mesh oxfords or "old lady shoes" of cordovan leather, Cuban heels and wing tips.

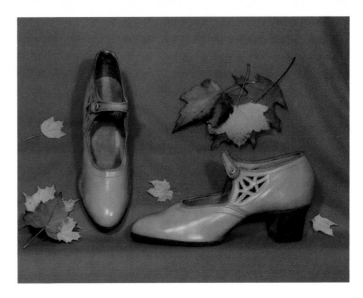

Beige leather shoes with geometric cutouts, buttoned straps, rounded toe, military heel.

CUTOUTS

The influences of Art Deco were ever present in the numerous geometric appliqués and metal ornaments. Ornate models with numerous geometric cutouts became the forerunners of the 1930s sandal.

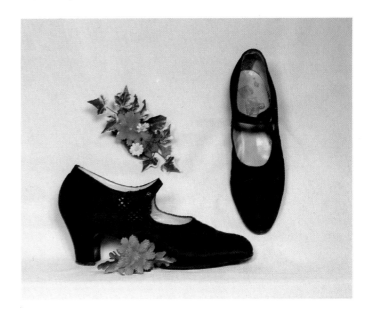

Black satin buttoned strap shoes, open grid at sides, Cuban heels. c. 1925-30 *Courtesy of Cedar Crest Alumnae Museum, gift of Ellie Laubner.*

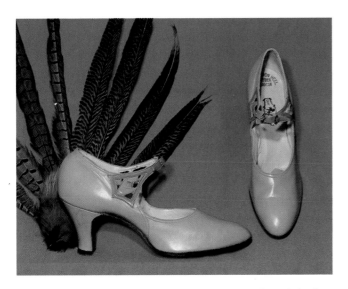

Tan leather shoes with Art Deco cutouts on straps, Spanish heels, c. mid-1920s. Marked: Sautter's, Utica, N.Y.

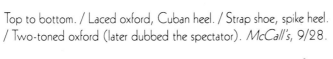

Top to bottom. / Laced oxford, Cuban heel. / Strap shoe, spike heel. / Two-toned oxford (later dubbed the spectator). *McCall's, 9/28.*

129

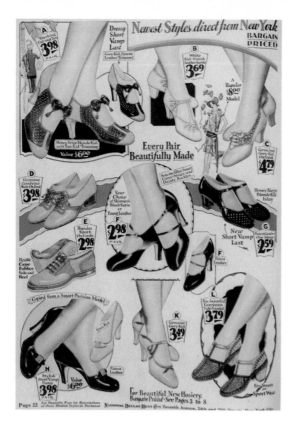

(A) a form of the Theo, (E) an early version of the saddle shoe, (L) the introduction of the huarache. National Bellas Hess Co., 1928. *Courtesy of Suzanjoy M. Checksfield.*

WORLD RENOWNED SHOE MAKERS

One of the finest shoe craftsman of the 1920s was Pietro Yantourny, an East Indian who worked in one of the chic shopping areas in Paris. Using exquisite fabrics and the finest leathers, he made elegant shoes of incomparable quality. According to Mary Trasko in her book *Heavenly Soles: Extraordinary 20th Century Shoes*, the sign in front of Yantourny's shop read "The world's most expensive custom shoemaker." He often required a $1,000 deposit on shoes which required up to two years to complete.

Other noted French shoe designers of the period were Charles Hellstern and André Perugia, who designed shoes for Paul Poiret. Alfred Argence's shoes graced the feet of European royalty as well as wealthy Americans.

Salvatore Ferragamo moved his shop from Florence to Hollywood in 1923, where he began designing shoes for early motion picture stars. Dissatisfied with the calibre of craftsmen in Hollywood, he returned to Florence in 1927, where he began exporting his elegant creations to prestigious stores in the United States.

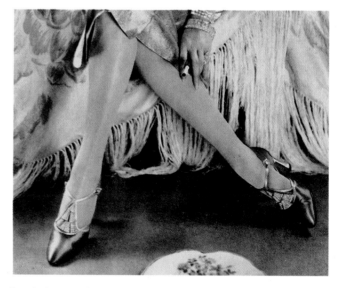

French designer shoes—green satin with Art Deco-style rhinestone ornaments by Perugia. *Vogue*, 10/25.

SPECTATORS

Also introduced at this time was the two-toned sport shoe, later called the spectator (known as a "co-respondent" in the U.K.). This white buckskin shoe had a contrasting quarter (back) and wing-tip (toe) of black, navy, or brown. Broguings were often placed along the edges of the dark leather.

HUARACHES

The 1929 Sears, Roebuck and Co. catalog advertised imported Mexican *huaraches* which were made of narrow closely woven strips of calfskin. They would become a favorite summertime sandal of the 1930s.

Added to the colors already mentioned were beige, parchment, sun tan, field mouse, light blue, rose blush, and honey blonde (light golden brown).

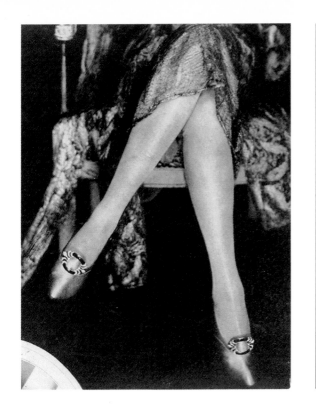

French designer pumps—blond satin with brown enamel and rhinestone ornaments by Hellstern. *Vogue*, 10/25.

NOTED SHOE MANUFACTURERS

A few of the noted shoe manufacturers of the 1920s were Cammeyer, Henning Cousins, Shoecraft, Delman, Slater, I. Miller, and Selby.

GALOSHES

During inclement weather men, women, and children wore rubber galoshes (boots) over their shoes. They featured two to six metal buckles which young girls preferred to leave open. This caused them to "flap-flap" as they walked, thus the name "flappers." The 1927-28 Charles William Stores catalog also advertised an overshoe with the new swift "slide fastener" (the zipper).

Boots with turned-down cuffs featured the new "jiffy fasteners" (zippers). / Black galoshes which were worn by flappers with the buckles open. Sears, Roebuck and Co., 1928-29.

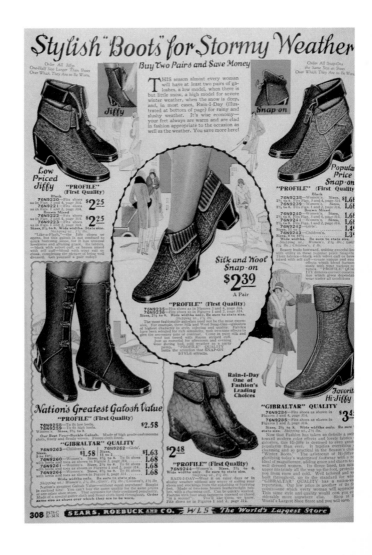

CHAPTER 11
JEWELRY

INFLUENCES

CHINESE

A taste for the exotic began during the preceding decade when the *Ballet Russe* (Russian Ballet) performed in Paris. The vibrant colors of the eastern costumes, designed by Léon Bakst, titillated the fashion-oriented French audiences. They also influenced French fashion designer Paul Poiret who dominated the fashion scene during the teens. This heightened interest in the East and lure for the exotic continued into the 1920s. Carved and pierced jade, carnelian, coral, cinnabar, ivory, and bone were all used in intriguing jewelry imported from China.

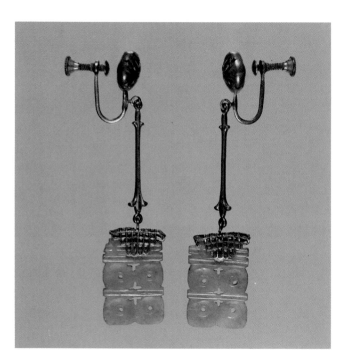

Oriental-style pendant earrings made of carved and pierced nephrite (a form of jade) and brass findings. *Courtesy of Ethel Bishop.*

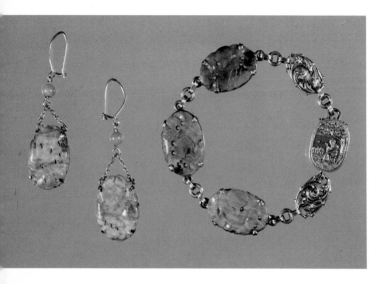

Chinese carved jade. / Pendant earrings. Marked: 10K. / Bracelet, sterling with gold wash. *Courtesy of Rose Jamieson.*

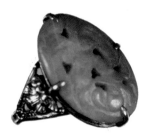

Carved and pierced nephrite ring in openwork setting. Marked: WL 14 K. *Courtesy of Ethel Bishop.*

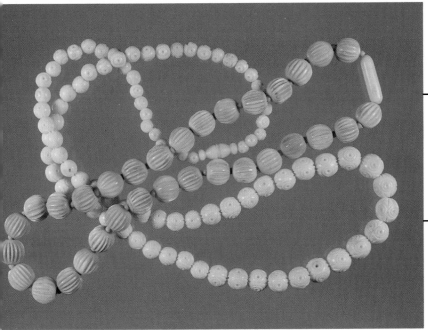

Carved bone necklaces. *Courtesy of Rose Jamieson.*

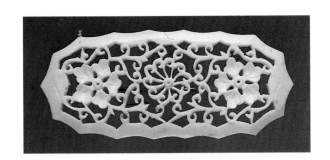

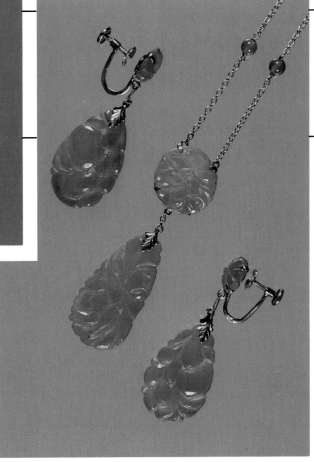

Chinese carved carnelian pendant and pendant earrings. Marked: 10K. *Courtesy of Rose Jamieson.*

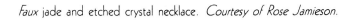

Two carved ivory brooches. *Courtesy of Rose Jamieson.*

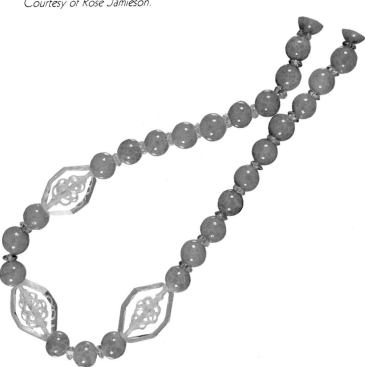

Faux jade and etched crystal necklace. *Courtesy of Rose Jamieson.*

EGYPTIAN

The treasure laden tomb of ancient Egyptian King Tutankhamen was discovered in 1922, the first such tomb to be found which had not been plundered by grave robbers. The discovery triggered a worldwide fascination with all things Egyptian. The spectacular objects found in the tomb inspired costume jewelry incorporating such motifs as the scarab, mummy, pharaoh, pyramid, obelisk, sphinx, vulture, asp, cobra, lotus, ankh (symbol of life), and hieroglyphics.

The most popular of these motifs was the scarab, a sacred Egyptian beetle. It was used alone or was substituted for the body of a falcon with outstretched wings. (Both the scarab and the falcon were symbols of the sun god Ra). Classic scarab bracelets were made of colored glass or semi-precious cabochons with engraved beetle markings. Scarab-style bracelets became popular again in the 1950s and 1960s.

Genuine or imitation lapis, turquoise, coral, and carnelian were used in making Egyptian-style pendants, bracelets, earrings, pins, and buckles.

Elaborate *parures* consisting of a bib-style fringed necklace, a wide multi-strand bracelet, and dangle earrings were very popular. These colorful sets were made with turquoise and coral colored glass beads or faience (a form of ceramic) with brass filigree findings.

Cuff, coiled serpent, or link-style "slave" bracelets were worn on the upper arm.

Necklace containing black molded glass resembling a Pharaoh, a mummy in coffin, Egyptian royalty, and winged scarab. (Missing 4-6 scarab beads.)

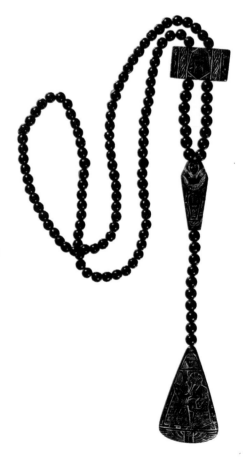

Scarab ring featuring engraved blood stone set in sterling Art Deco setting. Marked: sterling. *Courtesy of Rose Jamieson*

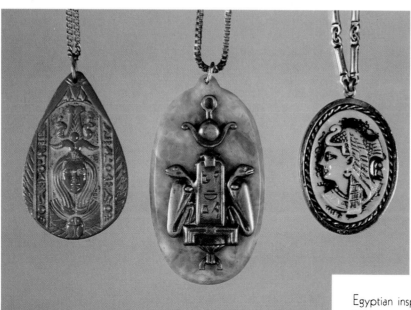

Egyptian inspired pendants. / Blue pressed-glass Pharaoh pendant. / Brass ornament on green bakelite oval. / Turquoise glass Pharaoh pendant. *Courtesy of Roseann Ettinger (Remember When…).*

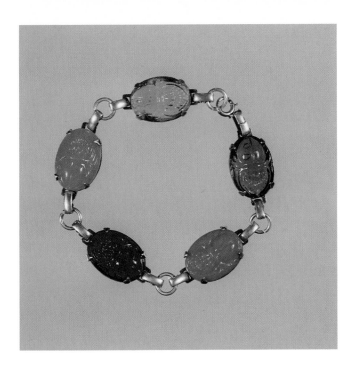

Pressed glass scarab bracelet set in sterling. Marked: sterling. *Courtesy of Suzanjoy M. Checksfield*

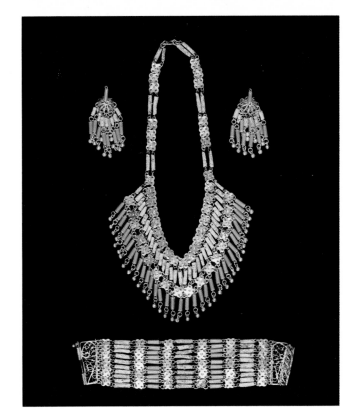

Dramatic Egyptian style demi-parure consisting of fringed earrings and necklace tipped with tiny round bells, plus a multi-strand bracelet. They were made from *faux* coral, blue *faience*, and brass filigree findings, c. 1924-1930.

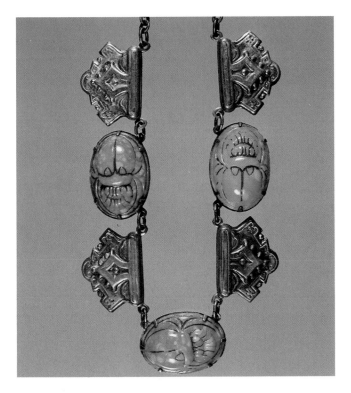

Scarab necklace of turquoise glass *cabochons* with beetle markings set in silver-plated brass links. *Courtesy of Roseann Ettinger (Remember When...).*

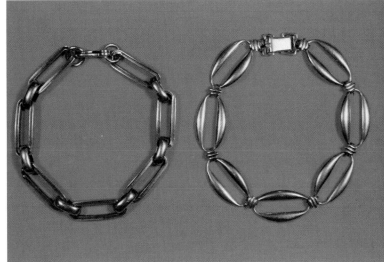

Silver-link slave bracelets which resemble chains of bondage. Marked: sterling. *Courtesy of Suzanjoy M. Checksfield*

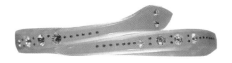

Egyptian-style celluloid snake bracelet with clear rhinestones and small pieces of cut steel, possibly worn on the upper arm.

ART DECO

In 1925, the *Parisian Exposition International des Arts Décoratifs et Industriels Modernes*, an international exhibit of modern decorative arts, was held in Paris. This display of decorative arts introduced to the world a new artistic style, which would later be called Art Deco. (See Chapter 1 for influences.)

Art Deco was characterized by geometric shapes, parallel lines, concentric circles, step patterns, sunbursts, waterfalls, fountains, stylized flowers, and other abstract motifs. These designs were frequently executed in a symmetrical format, i.e. "mirror-image" clasps, buckles, and hat ornaments.

Art Deco jewelry featured futuristic materials such as bakelite, chrome, and aluminum. Bakelite was the trade name for a phenolic resin (a form of plastic) invented in 1909 by Leo Hendrik Baekeland. It was initially produced to imitate more expensive natural substances such as ivory, tortoise shell, or amber. With the advent of Art Deco, however, people began to appreciate synthetic materials for their own unique qualities and the new and unusual effects which they could produce.

Dynamic color combinations such as black with red, white, silver, or Nile green were typical of Art Deco jewelry. The combinations of jet or onyx with crystal, marcasite, rhinestones, or diamonds were also prevalent.

WORLD RENOWNED ART DECO JEWELRY DESIGNERS

Cartier, Jean Fouquet, and Raymond Templier were three of the renowned designers of fine Art Deco jewelry.

Art Deco pendant watch on long *baton* link chain. (Reverse side) lovely *guilloché* enameling. (Front side) watch face with Art Deco-style numbers. Marked: sterling. *Courtesy of Rose Jamieson.*

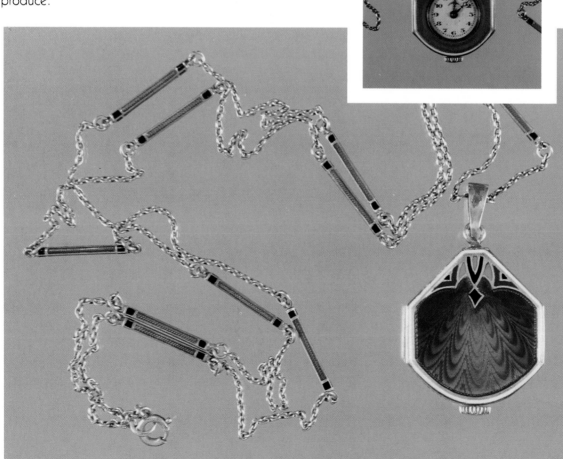

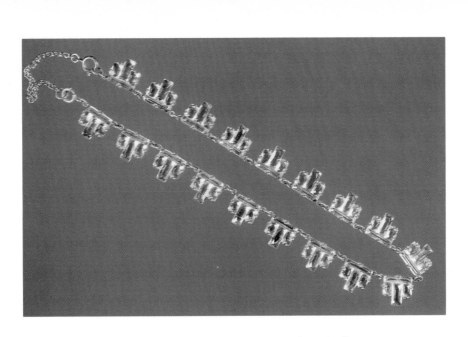

Clear rhinestone baguettes prong set in brass to form Art Deco step motif. c. 1925-1935.

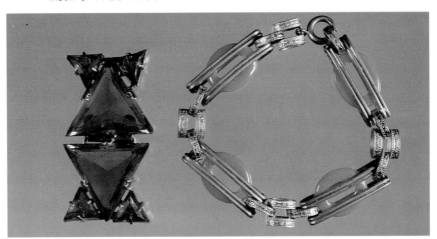

Green glass triangles prong set in Art Deco mirror-image buckle. / Gold-plated Art Deco bracelet with orange bakelite rings. *Courtesy of Roseann Ettinger (Remember When...).*

Art Deco-style novelty buckles. / Zinc setting with pavé set rhinestones and two bezel set triangular rhinestones. / Green rectangular rhinestones bezel set in brass. Marked: Czechoslovakia. c. late 20s-early 30s. *Courtesy of Suzanjoy M. Checksfield.*

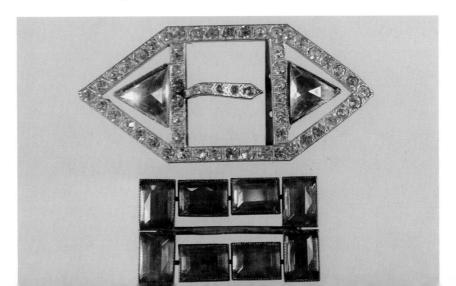

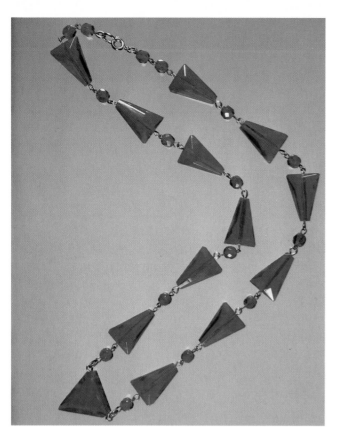

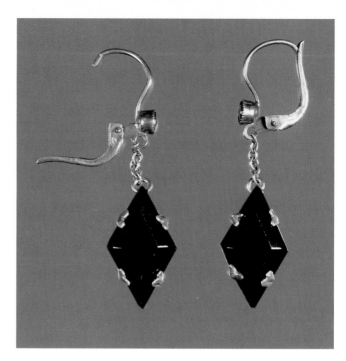

Diamond-shaped jet pendant earrings set in sterling silver with French lever-back ear wires. *Courtesy of Suzanjoy M. Checksfield.*

Red-faceted triangular and spherical glass beads strong on wire links. *Courtesy of Roseann Ettinger (Remember When...).*

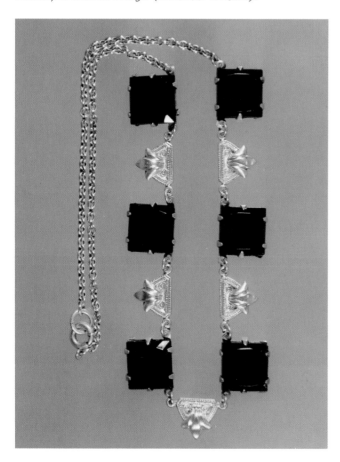

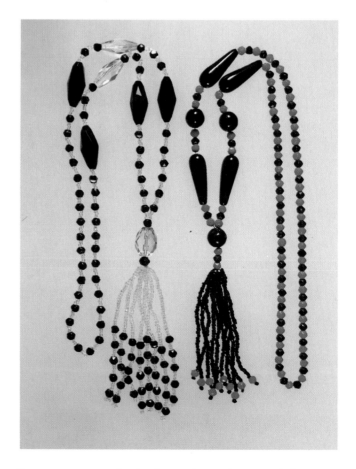

Squares of prong set black glass alternate with brass triangles to form this striking Art Deco necklace.

Two *sautoirs* in popular Art Deco color combinations. / Crystal and jet. *Courtesy of Grace Voorhees Howells.* / Red and black glass.

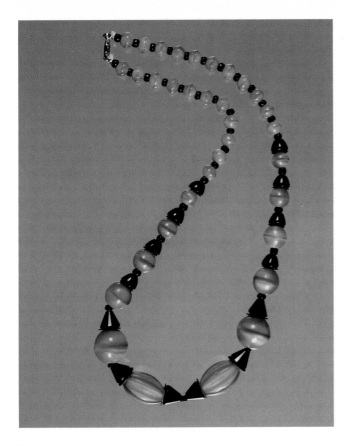

Short necklace of glass beads in popular Art Deco color combination.

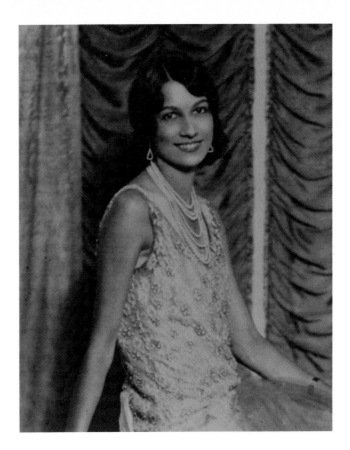

Flapper wearing drop earrings and multi-strand necklace of graduated pearls. *Courtesy of Rose Jamieson.*

MATERIALS

DIAMONDS

Due to the discovery of diamonds in the Kimberly fields of South Africa in 1866, diamonds became fashionable and more affordable. Dynamic color combinations were created by combining diamonds and onyx with rubies, emeralds, jade, or coral.

WHITE METALS

Because of its strength, white gold was used for setting precious stones, particularly diamonds. Its hardness made it ideal for the creation of delicate filigree jewelry which was so popular during the 1920s and 1930s. Its resemblance to highly-prized platinum also contributed to the shift from yellow gold to white gold.

Sterling silver, silver plate, nickel silver, and zinc were other metals used to imitate white gold in the production of less expensive jewelry.

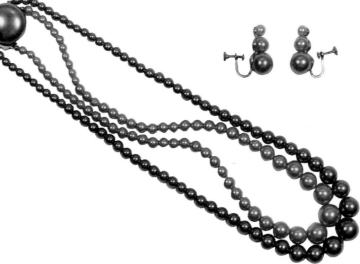

Imitation pearl necklace and screw-back earrings in two shades of olive green. *Courtesy of Suzanjoy M. Checksfield*

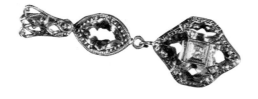

White gold filigree pendant with one square set diamond, five blue topaz stones. Marked: 14K. *Courtesy of Rose Jamieson.*

139

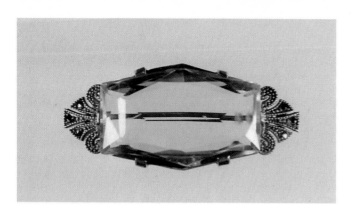

Pink glass brooch trimmed with marcasite. Marked: sterling. *Courtesy of Rose Jamieson.*

PEARLS

In 1915, a Japanese man by the name of Mikimoto perfected the process of cultivating cultured pearls. The less expensive cultured pearls drove down the prices of natural pearls as well. Pearl necklaces were a popular accessory worn for afternoon or evening. They came in single or multiple strands, the same or graduated sizes, and varying lengths. In general, longer strands were worn during the first half of the decade, while shorter necklaces became popular towards the end of the decade. Faux pearls were also tinted pastel pink, green, blue, and gray.

MARCASITE

Marcasite is an iron pyrite, first used in the 18th century as an inexpensive substitute for diamonds. It was opaque and therefore obtained its sparkle from the light reflected from its facets. Quality marcasite was prong set (not glued) into sterling silver jewelry. It was often combined with onyx for pendants, hair ornaments, necklaces, earrings, bracelets, rings, clasps, and hat ornaments. Imitation marcasite was produced by placing a silver coating over black glass stones.

Chrome-plated filigree pendant with faceted marquise-shaped rose crystal stone. *Courtesy of Roseann Ettinger (Remember When...).*

TECHNIQUES

STONE CUTS

Precious, semi-precious, and synthetic stones were cut primarily in geometric shapes including the emerald (rectangle), the baguette (narrow oblong), the tapered baguette (trapezoid), the lozenge (diamond), and the marquise (pointed oval).

FILIGREE

Filigree was extremely popular from the teens through the 1930s. It was used for pendants, bracelets, bar pins, earrings, rings, and circle pins. It was originally fashioned by hand from intricately twisted white gold or platinum wire, which was transformed into delicate openwork similar to lace. By the 1920s, however, filigree for semi-precious stones and costume jewelry was die cast from white gold, sterling silver, brass, nickel, and base metal. Within this lacy framework stones were set in square, rectangular, hexagonal, octagonal, and marquise-shaped settings.

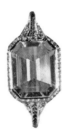

Gold filigree ring, blue topaz. Marked: 14K. *Courtesy of Rose Jamieson.*

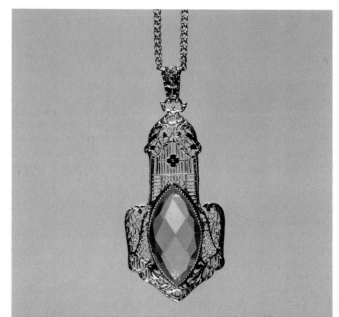

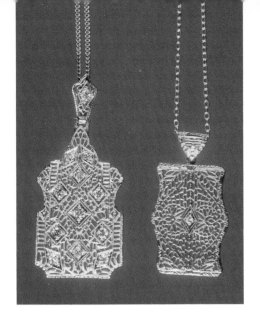

White gold filigree pendants. / Twelve diamonds in square settings. Marked: 14K. *Courtesy of Margaret Laubner Stish.* / Diamond in diamond-shaped setting. Marked: 10K. *Courtesy of Rose Jamieson.*

GUILLOCHÉ

Guilloché was a popular form of decoration for metal objects dating from the turn of the century through the 1930s. The object was first machine engraved in geometric all-over patterns called engine-turnings. Common patterns were sun rays; basket weaves; concentric circles; kaleidoscopes; and rows of dots, circles, squares, diamonds, waves, and stripes.

These engine-turnings were then covered with translucent enamel which allowed the engraved grooves to show through. Delicate pink roses, blue forget-me-nots, or baskets of flowers with blue ribbon bows were the dainty feminine designs most frequently hand painted over the *guilloché*. Finally an application of clear enamel was added as a protective coating.

STAR-CUT CRYSTAL

"Star-cut crystal" was a favorite form of jewelry during the 1920s and 1930s. The star burst motif was originally etched into a thin piece of rock crystal using acid or a cutting tool. A diamond was set into the center of the star and the crystal was then placed in a filigree pendant, bracelet, ring, or earrings. This process was executed on frosted glass, sometimes called "camphor glass" for a less expensive imitation of star-cut crystal.

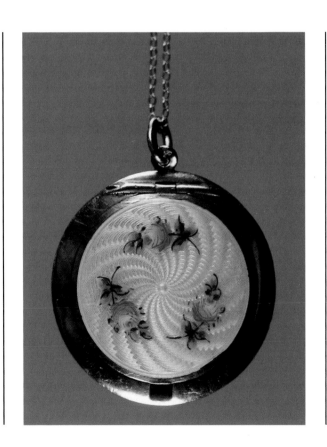

Silver locket with *guilloché* enameling in a pinwheel design and hand painted roses. Marked: Sterling. *Courtesy of Betty Teramo, inherited from Sophie Goetz.*

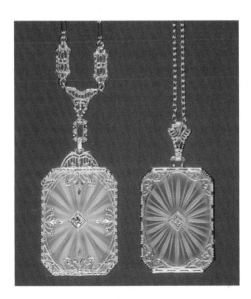

White gold filigree pendants containing star-cut crystal and square set diamonds. Both marked: 14K. *Left - Courtesy of Rose Jamieson.*

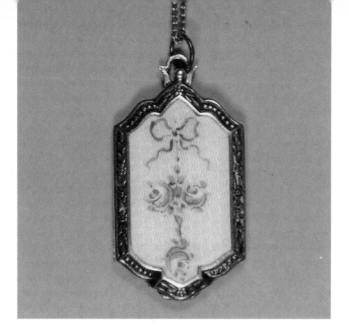

Sterling silver locket with hand-painted roses and blue ribbon over *guilloché* enameling. *Courtesy of Dolores Melkowits (Dee's Antiques).*

COSTUME JEWELRY

"Coco" Chanel introduced her "illusion jewelry" during the 1920s, which featured multiple strands of chain with imitation pearls and synthetic stones. It was an immediate success and soon even well-to-do women were decked in ostentatious jewelry with large synthetic stones.

JEWELRY FORMS

BEADED NECKLACES AND ROPES

Necklaces were made of transparent, translucent, and opaque glass beads in a myriad of geometric shapes and sizes. Although long 60-inch necklaces are more often associated with this period, shorter necklaces were also worn, particularly during the late twenties. These necklaces were so reasonable in price that even shop girls could afford to look stylish. In fact, it was common for women to purchase a necklace to coordinate with each outfit.

Many necklaces contained fancy Czechoslovakian "lampworked" beads. Each of these attractive beads was made by hand. Glass which contained gold stone (spangles of mica) was heated over a lamp, while pink molten glass was applied to the outer surface of the beads in tiny coils resembling rosebuds.

The necklace which is most representative of the period was the "*sautoir.*" It was made from various types of glass beads and ended with a long beaded tassel.

Flappers made their own *sautoirs* (similar to those made by the American Indians) by weaving *rocaille* (seed beads) on small hand looms. Bead companies printed patterns for these *sautoirs* which were often referred to as "flapper beads."

Crocheted ropes were made of seed beads, accented on either end with Czechoslovakian lampworked beads and beaded tassels. The ends could be flipped over one another, or the rope could be worn hacking style around the neck. (See illustration.)

Necklaces made of wood and paper maché beads were also popular throughout the 1920s and 1930s.

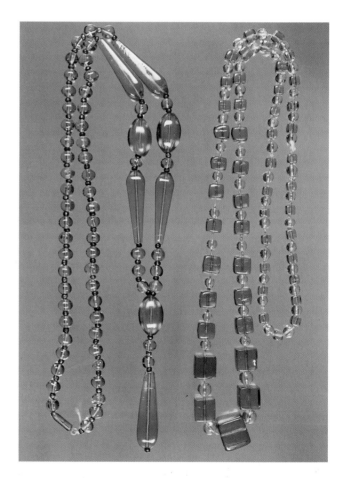

Necklaces of geometric-shaped amber glass beads.

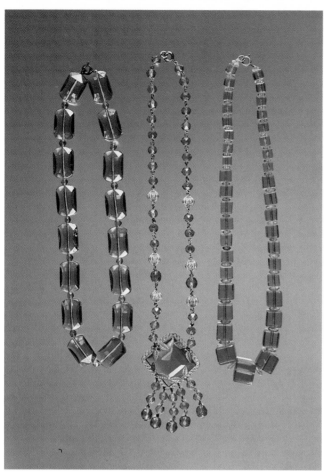

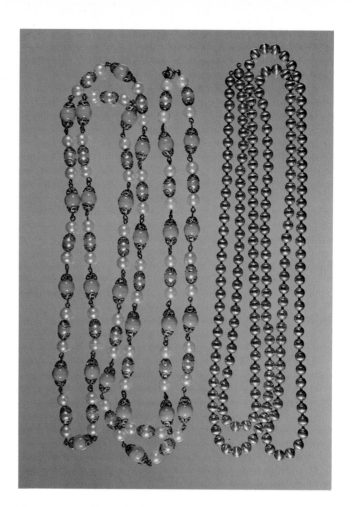

Three necklaces of geometric blue glass beads, center has silver-plated filigree beads and pendant. *Courtesy of Roseann Ettinger (Remember When...).*

Waist-length necklace of light green glass beads, pearls, and brass filigree strung on brass wire links. / Brass ball-chain necklace.

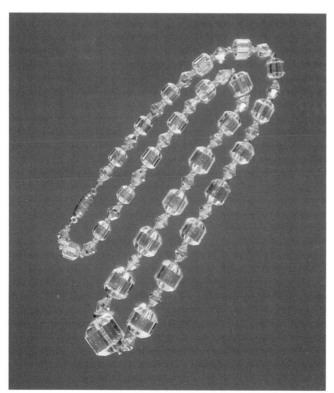

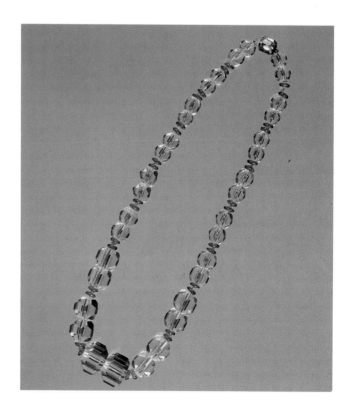

Necklace of crystal beads and brass spacers. *Courtesy of Rose Jamieson.*

Necklace of faceted graduated clear glass beads with green stripes and green glass rondelles. *Courtesy of Theresa Schouten.*

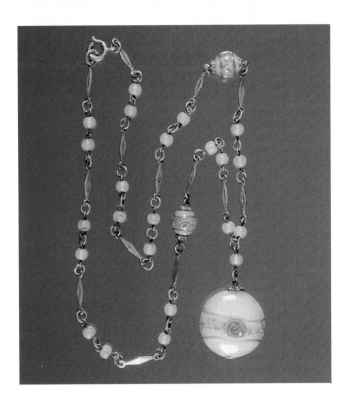

Necklace of yellow Czechoslovakian glass lampworked beads containing goldstone and pink rosebud trim.

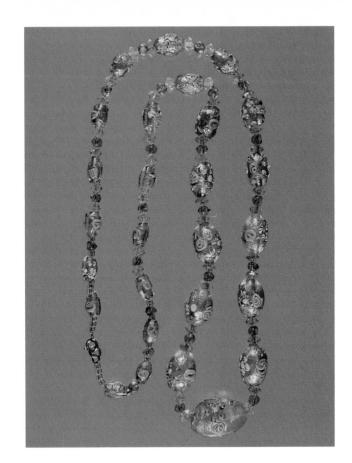

Necklace of Czechoslovakian glass lampworked beads with rosebud trim. *Courtesy of Rose Jamieson.*

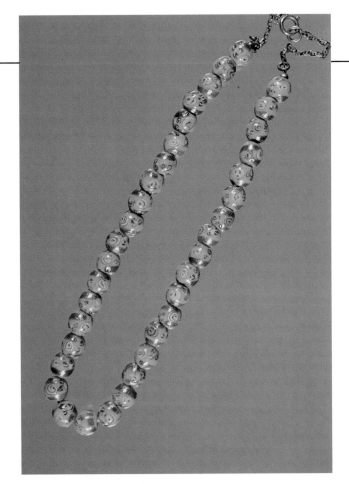

Turquoise necklace of Czechoslovakian glass lampworked beads with rosebud and goldstone trim. *Courtesy of Rose Jamieson.*

Necklace of pink molded glass and white Czechoslovakian glass lampworked beads with blue and gold enamel and rosebud trim.

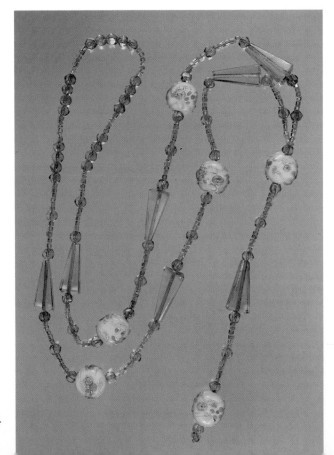

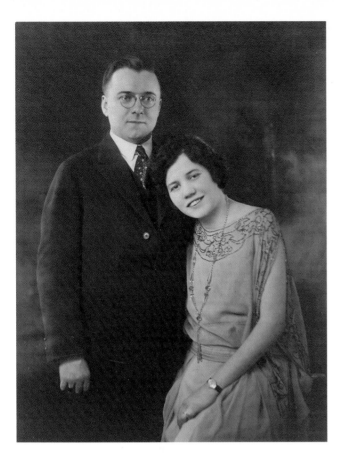

Woman wearing long *sautoir* over beaded dress with boat-neck. Man wears *pince-nez* eyeglasses and suit with high lapels, c. early 1920s.

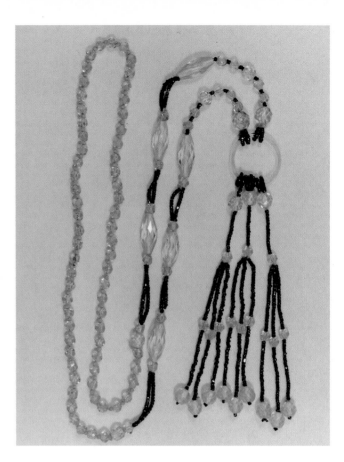

Waist-length *sautoir* of yellow faceted glass beads and black iridescent seed beads.

Waist-length *sautoir* of turquoise faceted glass beads.

Delicate waist-length *sautoir* of green and black glass beads strong on fine curb chain with beaded tassel.

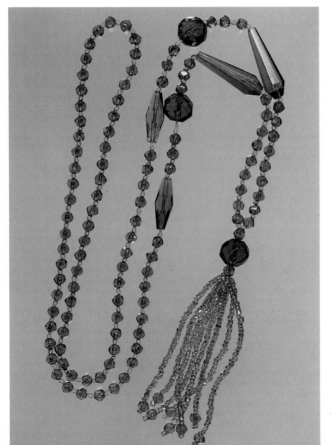

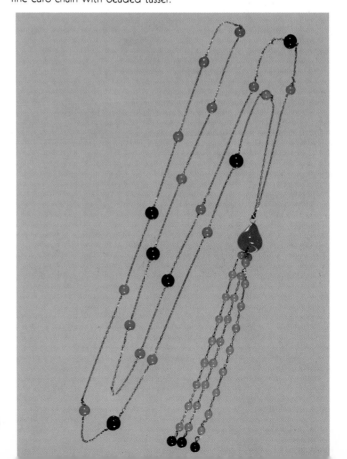

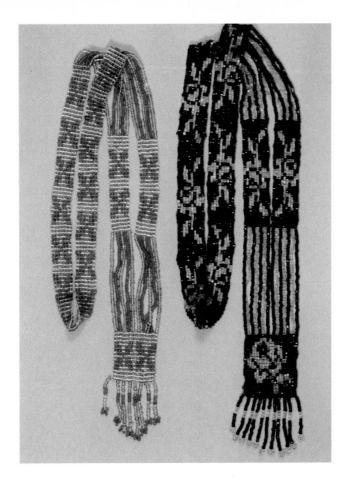

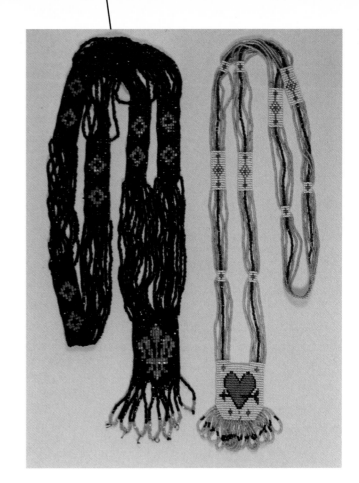

Two *sautoirs*. / X motif, deep red and silver colored seed beads. / Rose motif, black and opalescent seed beads.

Two *sautoirs*. / Unusual red, green, gold, and blue carnival glass seed beads. / Black and gold seed beads with wearer's initials (JH), beaded loop fringe.

Two *sautoirs*. / Red fleur-de-lis and diamonds with black seed beads. / Red heart and diamonds on blue and white seed beads. *Courtesy of Suzanjoy M. Checksfield.*

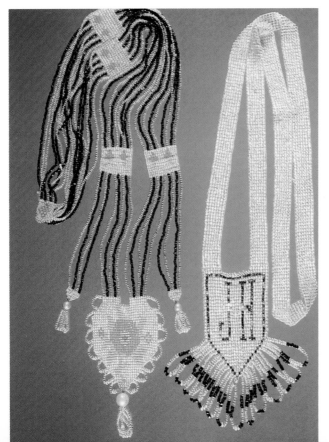

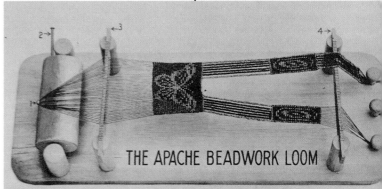

THE APACHE BEADWORK LOOM

Apache brand beadwork loom for making seed bead *sautoirs*.

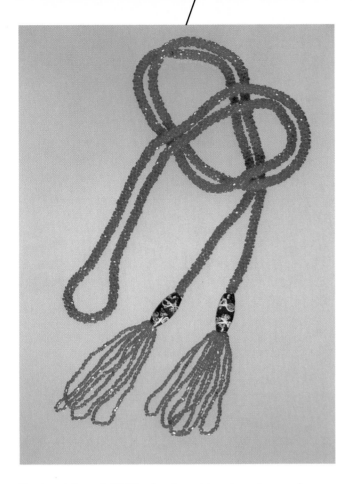

Crocheted "rope" (54") of red seed beads with two decorative Czechoslovakian glass lampworked beads containing goldstone and rosebud trim.

EARRINGS

Pendant earrings with single or multiple dangles were all the rage. Earrings contained either screw backs or wires for pierced ears.

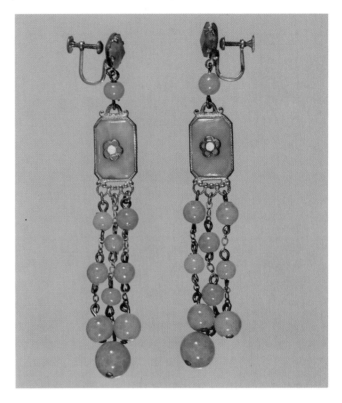

Green glass dangle earrings with brass screw-back fittings.

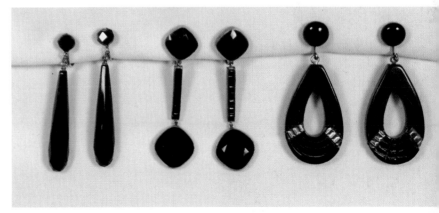

Black screw-back Art Deco pendant earrings. / Faceted spheres and drops. / Four bezel set squares of faceted glass, smaller channel set squares. Marked: sterling. / Dangling loops of black bakelite with parallel ridges. *Courtesy of Suzanjoy M. Checksfield*

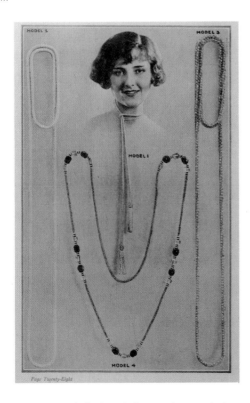

Suggested way to wear the beaded rope along with three additional necklaces. *Hiawatha Beaded Bags and Chains* (instruction booklet), 1924. *Courtesy of Rose Jamieson.*

BRACELETS

Filigree bracelets in flexible or bangle styles were decorated with precious and semi-precious stones. Sterling silver bracelets adorned with marcasite were produced in link and bangle styles. Inexpensive celluloid bangles were decorated with colored rhinestones. Towards the end of the decade, dynamic Art Deco bracelets were made of modernistic materials such as bakelite, chrome, and aluminum.

Several bracelets were frequently worn at a time, often on the upper arm. This was possible because of the vogue for sleeveless evening dresses.

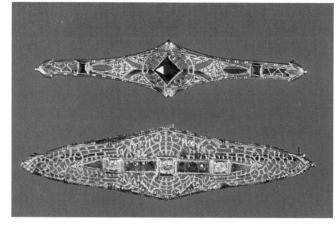

White gold filigree bar pins. / Three sapphires. Marked: 14K. / Eight emeralds, three diamonds. Marked: 10K. *Courtesy of Rose Jamieson*

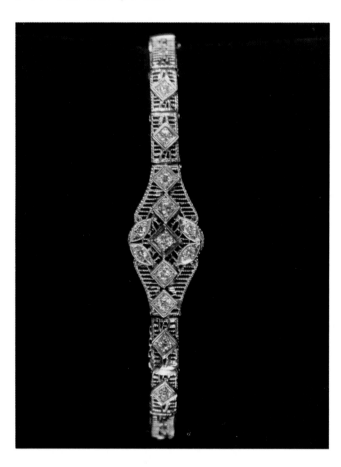

White gold filigree segmented bracelet with thirteen diamonds in square and marquise-shaped settings. *Courtesy of Margaretha J. Laubner*

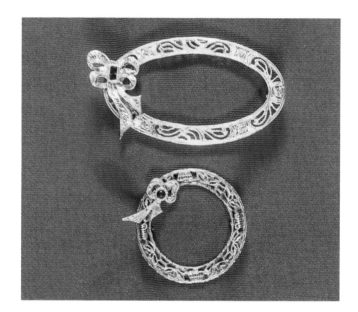

White gold filigree circle pins with ribbon bows. / Sapphires and diamonds. Marked: 14K. / Sapphire *cabochon*. Marked: 10K. *Courtesy of Rose Jamieson.*

Filigree bracelet, one marquise-shaped aquamarine, four diamonds. Marked: platinum top. *Courtesy of Rose Jamieson.*

148

BROOCHES

Filigree bar, circle, and oval pins were popular, as well as brooches featuring large geometric stones. Bowknot pins, inspired by the diamond ribbon brooches worn by England's Queen Mary, were popular throughout the 1920s.

The classic cameo remained in style. Stone and shell cameos were carved with characteristically plump maidens bedecked with flowers. There was often a geometric-shaped diamond pendant hanging from a very fine chain around the maiden's neck.

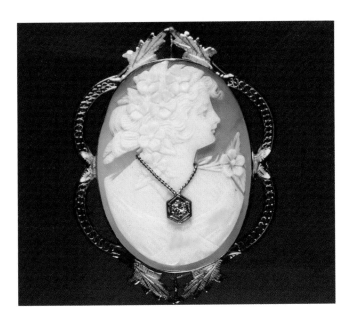

Italian shell cameo brooch/pendant, white gold filigree frame, diamond in hexagonal setting. Marked: 14K. *Courtesy of Margaretha J. Laubner.*

RINGS

Filigree was used extensively for rings during the 1920s and 1930s. Birthstone and cameo rings were popular, as well as rings containing onyx with a diamond or an initial centerpiece.

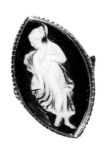

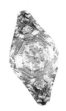

White gold filigree ring, center diamond set in hexagon. Marked: 18K. *Courtesy of Rose Jamieson.*

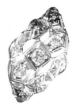

White gold ring with five diamonds. Marked: 18K. *Courtesy of Rose Jamieson.*

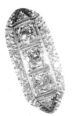

Platinum ring, five diamonds surrounded by *pavè* set diamond chips. *Courtesy of Rose Jamieson.*

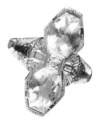

White gold filigree ring, two hexagonal aquamarine, diamond center. Marked: 14K. *Courtesy of Rose Jamieson.*

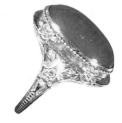

Gold filigree rings. / *Faux* sapphire surrounded by pearls, raised ribbon bows at sides. Marked: 14K. / Carnelian *cabochon*, channel for pearls (missing) with flower blossoms. Marked: 14K. *Courtesy of Rose Jamieson.*

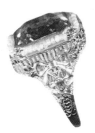

Gold ring with marquise-shaped stone cameo. Marked: 14K. *Courtesy of Rose Jamieson.*

WATCHES

Watches featured elaborately engraved frames in geometric shapes including the square, marquis, barrel, octagon, hexagon, and rectangle. They were made primarily of platinum, white gold, or sterling. Art Deco-style numbers were often used on watch faces. Watches were offered with black grosgrain or flexible metal bands. Elegant filigree watch/bracelets were designed to be worn on either the handsome watch side, or the attractive jeweled bracelet side. Pendant watches were often enameled with attractive Art Deco motifs. It was common for the watch stem to be set with a sapphire or blue glass cabochon similar to those which adorned the clasps of handbag frames.

NOTED WATCH MAKERS

A few of the more prominent watch makers were: Gruen, Elgin, Hamilton, Bulova, and Movado.

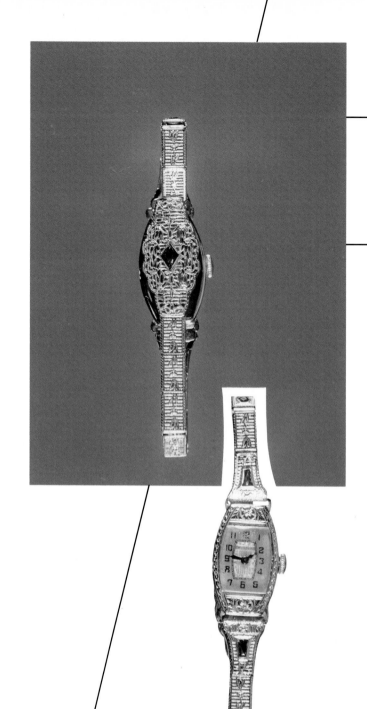

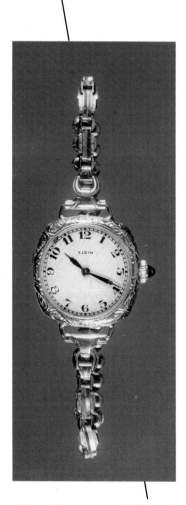

Reversible white gold filigree watch/bracelet (can be worn on either side). Marked: Bulova 14K. *Courtesy of Rose Jamieson.*

Engraved white gold watch, stem set with blue *cabochon*. Marked: Elgin 14K. *Courtesy of Rose Jamieson.*

150

CHAPTER 12
ACCESSORIES AND RELATED ITEMS

EYEGLASSES

OVAL FRAMES

In the late teens and early 1920s, eyeglass rims began to change in shape from oval to round. A look at the eyeglasses pictured in any college yearbook of the mid-1920s reveals that many of the professors were still clinging to outdated oval lenses (with or without rims). Conservative professors even preferred the "*pince-nez*" (pinch nose) style which had no temples. They were held precariously on the bridge of the nose by spring-tension nose pads.

ROUND TORTOISE FRAMES

Students, on the other hand, embraced the genuine or simulated tortoise-shell eyeglasses with round rims. These dark frames became the trademark of 1920s comedian Harold Lloyd. Other round eyeglass frames of the 1920s were made of 14K white gold, or were gold-plated or gold filled. The rims of these glasses were often decorated with raised border designs.

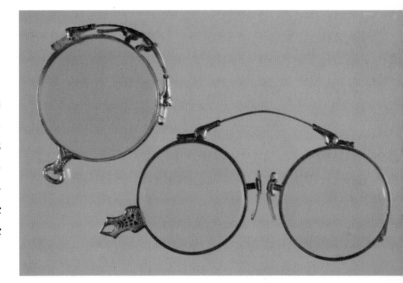

Folding Oxford *pince-nez* glasses, frame engraved with border of Art Deco sunrays. / Folded specs. Marked: Schwab PAT. 2/24/22, 12K 1/10 TxP. / Open specs. Marked: 14K SPG. *Courtesy of Dr. Benson Olenick.*

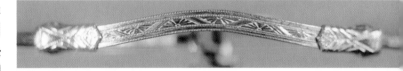

Top view of nose bridge with typical raised Art Deco sunray design. *Courtesy of Dr. Benson Olenick*

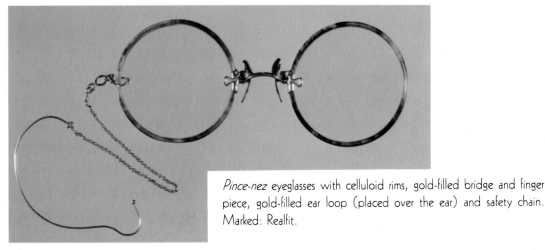

Pince-nez eyeglasses with celluloid rims, gold-filled bridge and finger piece, gold-filled ear loop (placed over the ear) and safety chain. Marked: Realfit.

EYEGLASS MANUFACTURERS

Some of the major eyeglass manufacturers of the period included: Bausch and Lomb, Realfit, Schwab, Shur-on, Optical Products Corporation, American Optical Company, and Stoco.

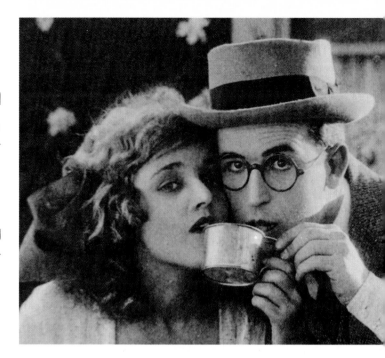

Lobby card promoting the movie *Grandma's Boy* (1922) staring Harold Lloyd, the 1920s comedian. He wears the round dark-rimmed eyeglasses which became his trademark.

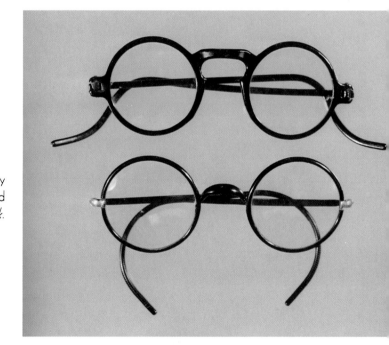

Round "Harold Lloyd" style eyeglasses. / Black phenolic resin, early split joint hinges. / Brass core covered with phenolic resin, gold-filled hinges. Marked: G.F. SHUR-ON. *Courtesy of Dr. Benson Olenick.*

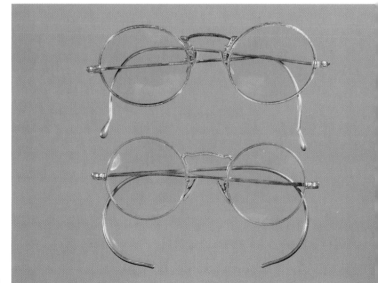

Engraved white gold-filled eyeglass frames with round rims. Top pair, marked: B&L (Bausch & Lomb). *Courtesy of Margaretha J. Laubner.*

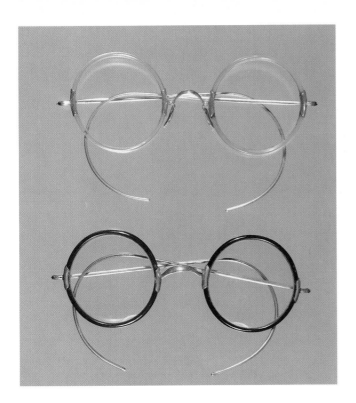

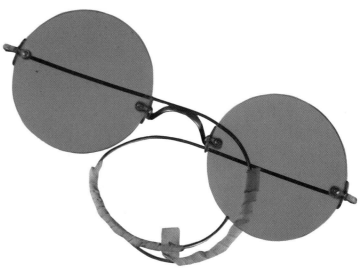

Round yellow/green glass lenses, cable temples wrapped with cloth tape. Marked: Eclipses Protection Glasses on box. Possibly used to view solar eclipse in 1923 or 1925. *Courtesy of Dr. Benson Olenick.*

Celluloid circular rims; gold-filled bridges, and cable temples. / Marked: MO Co. / Marked: STOCO 1/10-12K. *Courtesy of Dr. Benson Olenick.*

GLOVES

Long white kid or chamoisette gloves with buttons at the wrist were worn with formal evening wear. Short gloves of silk, charmeuse, kid, suede, doeskin, and felted cotton were worn with fashionable afternoon attire. They were offered in neutral colors such as brown, beige, tan, gray, black, and white, or they were dyed to match a particular outfit.

These short daytime gloves developed a small cuff which was often decorated with perforations, appliqués or embroidery. Some gloves had a pleated or gathered ruffle at the wrist which could be turned up or down, as desired. These cuffed gloves were well on their way to becoming the "gauntlet" or "*mousquetaire*" gloves of the 1930s, named for the gauntlets with flared cuffs worn by musketeers of the 17th century.

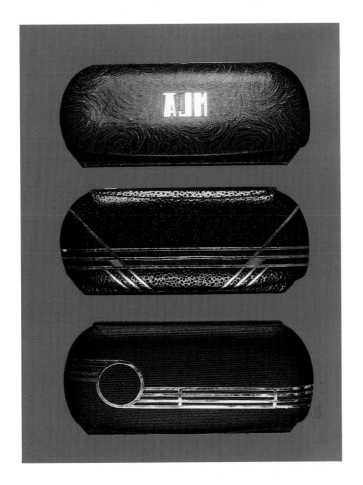

Three steel "frog mouth" eyeglass cases decorated with Art Deco initials and parallel aluminum strips. *Courtesy of Margaretha J. Laubner.*

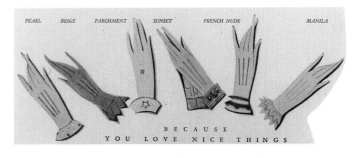

Gloves with small cuffs by Van Raalte. *McCall's, summer 1927.*

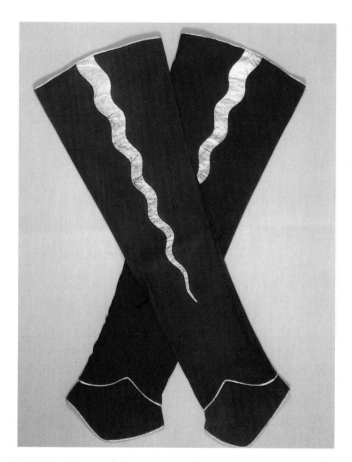

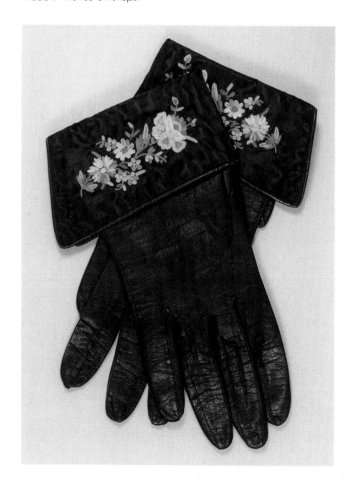

Ivory kid gloves with embroidery, geometric appliqués on cuffs. Marked: Made in France on snaps.

MAKERS OF FINE GLOVES

Firms noted for their fine gloves were Van Raalte, Alexandre, and Perrault.

High-fashion brown suede fingerless mitts with gold leather trim. Marked: Made Expressly for Neiman Marcus Co. US PAT Sept. 19 '22. *Courtesy of Pauline Laubner Burleson.*

Black rayon novelty gloves with monkey fur trim. Made minor sensation when worn with black dress to college dance, 1927. *Courtesy of Mildred Boitano.*

Black kid gloves with polychromatic *tambour* embroidery. Marked: *Point de Beauvain, Au Printemps* 2403 Paris.

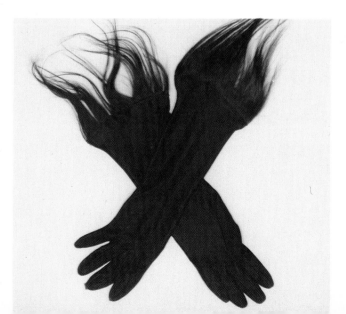

154

UMBRELLAS AND PARASOLS

UMBRELLAS

In 1924, the long thin umbrellas of the previous two decades were replaced by short "modish stub-shaped" models with 8-24 ribs. The thick, often carved handles, rib tips, and stub ends were made of ivory, horn, ebony, amber colored celluloid, bakelite, or wood. Attached to the handle was a braided silk-cord wrist loop which ended in a large bead or tassel. The silk, cotton, and rayon taffeta covers were primarily decorated with contrasting borders, concentric stripes, or geometric motifs.

PARASOLS

Parasols were still used as protection from the sun for afternoon outings, garden parties, and visits to the seaside. They also became short and stubby during the later half of the decade. (See Chapter 6 for a description.)

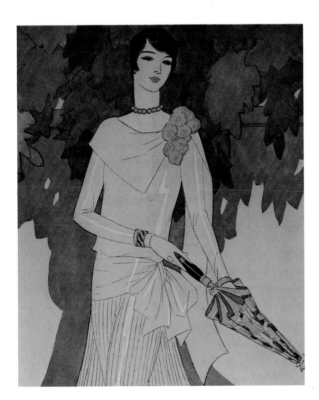

Typical short stubby parasol in popular 20s colors. *Fashion Service Magazine*, May 1928. *Courtesy of Suzanjoy M. Checksfield*

FANS

FASHION FANS

The days of the fabulous fashion fan were numbered. Fans were now carried more as a decorative accessory for evening wear than a cooling device. They were primarily made of plumes or feathers in the fashionable colors of the decade or dyed to match a particular gown. Ostrich plumes were fashioned into long fans with only one to three sticks. A wider, more dramatic-style fan was made of curved feathers all sweeping in the same direction.

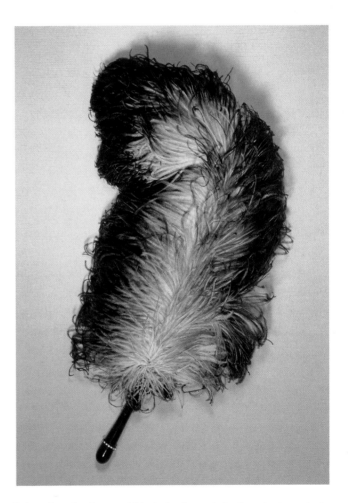

Fashion fan of yellow and black dyed ostrich feather plumes with *faux* tortoise shell handle, decorative silver ring contains seventeen rose point diamonds. *Courtesy of Wendy Hamilton Blue.*

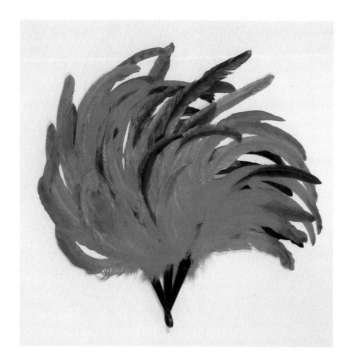

Dramatic Art Deco fashion fan of red and black curved feathers, three dark brown celluloid sticks.

ADVERTISING FANS

While fashion fans were dwindling in number, paper advertising fans were experiencing a heyday. These inexpensive but attractive fans were cleverly employed as promotional handouts. Some fans were given as souvenirs of places or events, while others were used to promote political candidates. Fans with photos of the latest film stars were distributed at movie theaters as a means for keeping cool. *Couture* houses and department stores advertised clothing, accessories, perfumes, and cosmetics by the use of advertising fans. There were two primary varieties, the flat fan which was mounted on a wooden stick, and the folding fan which was produced in both the "balloon" and the "*fontange*" (shell) shape.

Advertising fan featuring female stars of Paramount Pictures. Note: Clara Bow and Louise Brooks. c. early 1920s. *Courtesy of Wendy Hamilton Blue.*

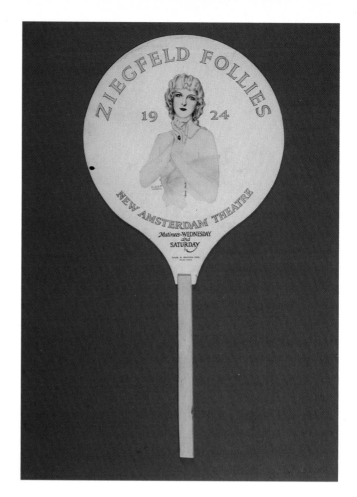

Cardboard advertising fan given to patrons for their comfort at the New Amsterdam Theater, features Ziegfeld Follies ad designed by Albert Vargas, 1924. *Courtesy of Wendy Hamilton Blue.*

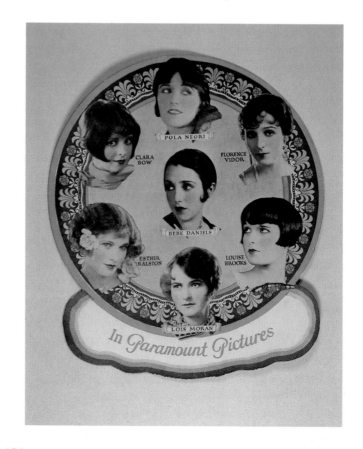

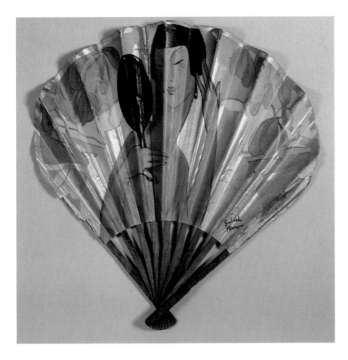

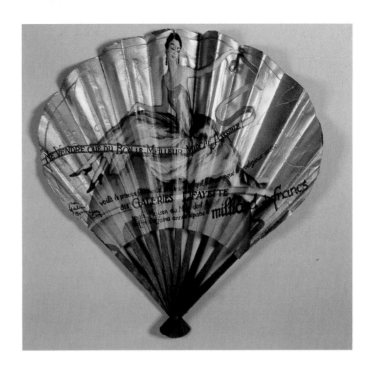

Galeries Lafayette advertising fan. (Front view) Oriental woman with bobbed hair, designed by Gabriel Ferro. *Courtesy of Wendy Hamilton Blue.*

Galeries Lafayette fan. (Back view) Women sitting on top of the world, designed by Jean Gabriel Domerque. Marked: France 1926.

NOTED FAN ILLUSTRATORS

Many attractive advertising fans were designed by renowned artists and fashion illustrators of the period such as Raoul Dufy, Paul Iribe, George Barbier, Georges Lepape, Fernand Couderc, Guy-Pierre Fauconnet, Jean Gabriel Domergue, Edouard Malouze, J. Ganne, Jack Roberts, Marcel Guelain, and Gabriel Ferro.

DANCE PROGRAMS

Dancing was an extremely popular pastime during the 1920s. Formal attire was usually required for evening affairs, while fancy day dresses and hats were worn to afternoon "tea dances."

Dance programs were issued to each young lady either prior to, or at a dance. Each program contained a column of numbers (i.e. one to ten) which corresponded to the number of dances scheduled for the affair. (A dance consisted of four or five songs.) An intended male partner could reserve a dance with a young lady by signing her dance program beside the number of his choice. The dance program then served as a memory aid for the participants. A girl generally saved the first and the last dance for the young man who escorted her to the affair.

Dance programs were usually made of good quality paper or artificial leather. Celluloid covers were a bit more costly and were, therefore, reserved for special occasions. A tiny pencil was often attached with a silk cord. When the dance was over, the program served as a souvenir of the event and was proudly hung on the mirror above the young lady's bureau.

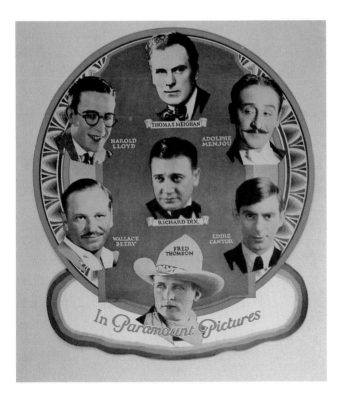

Advertising fan featuring male stars of Paramount Pictures. Note: Harold Lloyd in tortoise-shell glasses. 1927. *Courtesy of Wendy Hamilton Blue.*

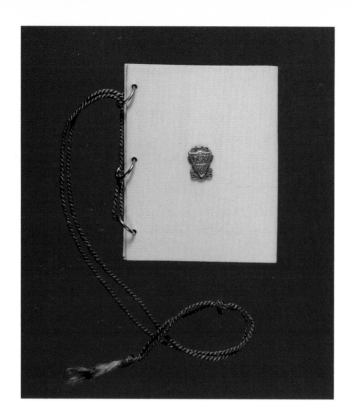

Loose-leaf dance program, celluloid cover with brass fraternity crest. Inside reads: Pi Chapter of Kappa Delta, February 3, 1923, numbers "one-ten."

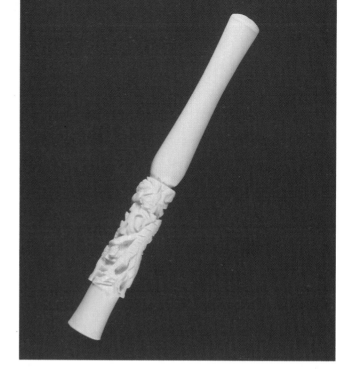

Ivory cigarette holder hand carved with Oriental dragon. Style popular teens-1950s.

SMOKING ACCESSORIES

Smoking doubled during the 1920s which created a demand for cigarette holders, cases, and lighters. These smoking accessories could be purchased separately or in attractive matching sets. Cigarette holders were generally made of amber, ivory, or colorful nonflammable bakelite.

Cigarette cases and lighters were made of sterling, brass, nickel silver, or base metal. They were plated with gold, silver, nickel, or chrome. The favorite forms of decoration for these items were hand and machine engraving, hammering, embossing, enameling, *guilloché, cloisonné*, leather, and alligator or snakeskin. After 1925, bold geometric Art Deco designs were applied to chrome-plated accessories in dynamic color combinations such as black with red, white, or green.

Monogramming was extremely popular during the 1920s. A smooth *cartouche* (usually rectangular during the 1920s) was often provided on metal objects for the engraving of ones initials.

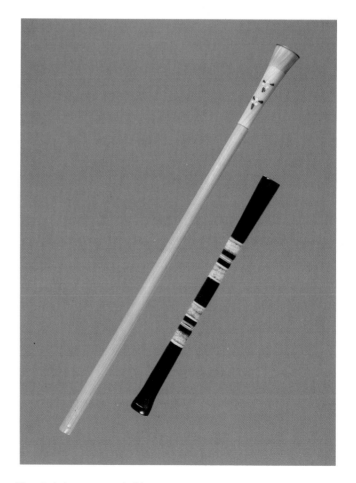

Two bakelite cigarette holders.

158

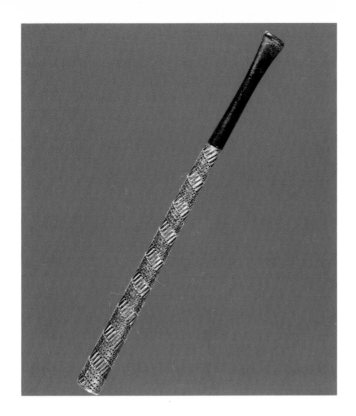

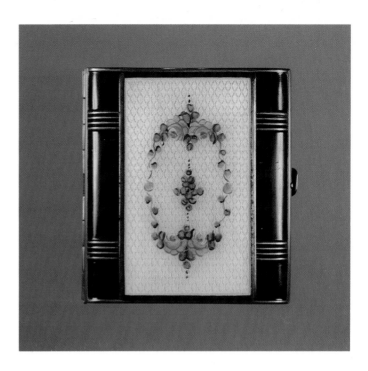

Cigarette holder, intricate silver spiral design over brass core, bakelite mouth piece. *Courtesy of Richard Groman.*

Silver-plated brass cigarette case with hand-painted flowers over *guilloché* enameling. Marked: La Mode. *Courtesy of Theresa Schouten.*

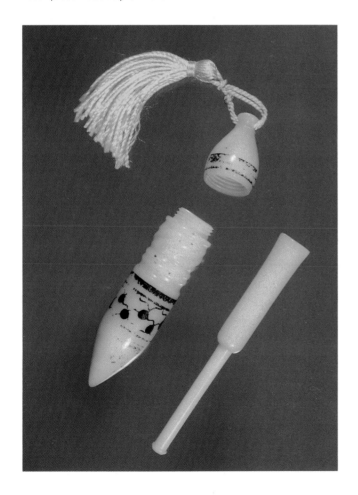

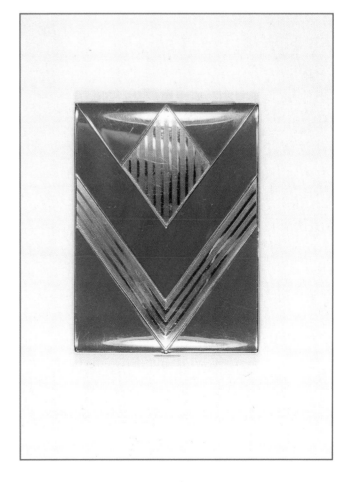

For the women on the go, a mini bakelite telescoping cigarette holder which fits neatly into the handy capsule. Marked: Germany.

Chrome-plated cigarette case with green enameled Art Deco design and engine-turnings, c.1925-35.

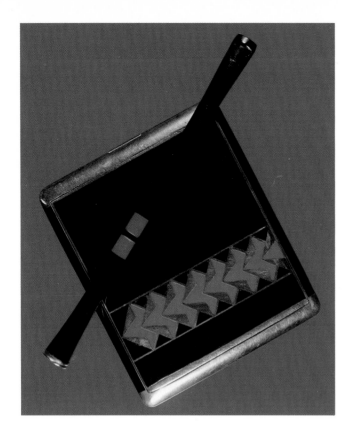

Deliciously Deco chrome-plated cigarette case with red and black enameled geometric design. *Courtesy of Richard Groman.* Red and black bakelite cigarette holder.

DRINKING ACCESSORIES

Prohibition went into effect in 1920, but instead of solving the alcohol problem in this country, it turned drinking into a national pastime. When drinking became illegal, people devised ingenious ways of concealing the "hooch" in their clothing or accessories. Photographs in the *Time and Life* series called "*This Fabulous Century: 1920-1930*" show flasks hidden in a cane handle, a boot, and a ladies' garter.

Chrome-plated "hip flasks" came into popular use for men in the early 1920s. They were slightly curved to fit the contours of a man's back pocket. Flasks were hammered, engraved, or covered with leather. Small rectangular *cartouches* were also placed on flasks for engraved initials.

Small flasks for women were designed to be carried in a pocket or purse. Quality flasks were made of sterling silver or cut glass.

Men's small hammered-metal hip flask with *cartouche* for monogram, chrome finish (2 3/4" x 3").

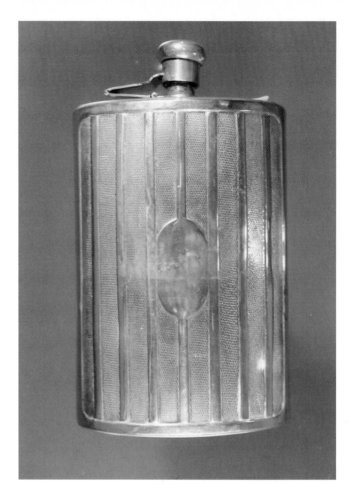

Men's chrome-plated hip flask with *cartouche* for monogram. *Courtesy of Elaine Cruse.*

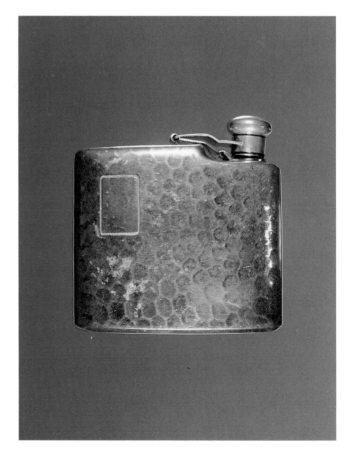

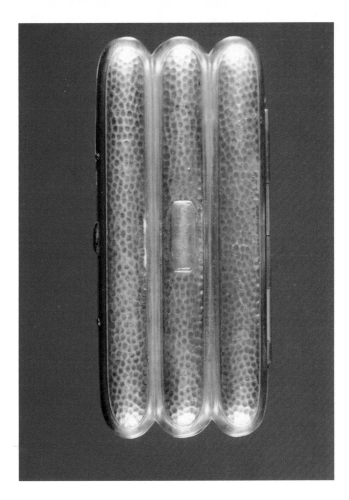

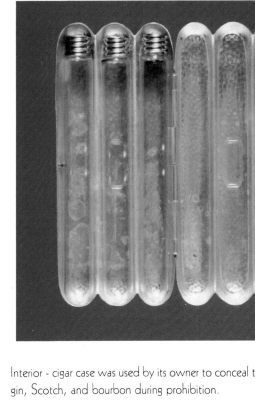

Interior - cigar case was used by its owner to conceal three glass vials for gin, Scotch, and bourbon during prohibition.

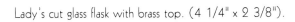

Exterior - hammered aluminum cigar case with monogram *cartouche*.

Lady's cut glass flask with brass top. (4 1/4" x 2 3/8").

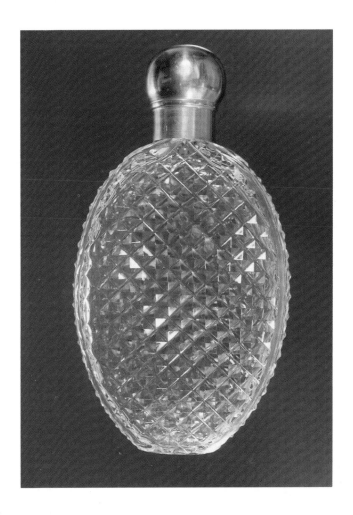

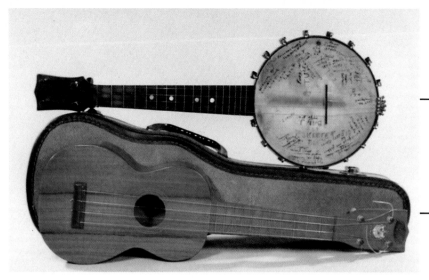

Ukulele banjo signed by flapper's friends, class of 1920. / Ukulele used by another flapper in High School orchestra, 1920s. Marked: Paul Summers Famous Waikiki Ukulele, Tabu Made in Honolulu. *Courtesy of Theresa Schouten.*

LUGGAGE

Paid vacations and newer, more rapid modes of transportation encouraged many people to travel. Whether traveling by ship or by rail, the wardrobe trunk was an indispensable companion. These trunks were made with numerous specialized compartments to organize the traveler's wardrobe and "store dresses, suits, and accessories without wrinkling." Students found these trunks handy for transporting clothing to and from college.

The most prestigious name in handcrafted luggage of the period was Louis Vuitton of Paris. The intertwined LV trademark stood for a firm with an "established reputation for responding to the demands of the most sophisticated travelers."

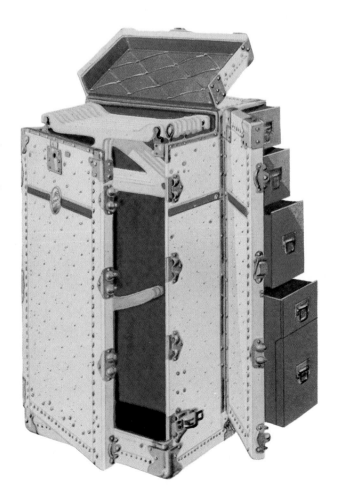

Winship wardrobe trunk equipped with hangers and drawers. *Vogue,* 1926.

CHAPTER 13

MEN'S WEAR

Styles for men changed much slower than styles for women. In fact, many of the garments mentioned in this chapter had been worn by men since the Victorian era.

Just as stylish women looked to Paris for trends in women's fashion, the well-dressed male looked to London (Bond Street and Savile Row) for the latest in men's wear styles. The Prince of Wales (Duke of Windsor), considered by many to be the arbiter of men's fashion, introduced many styles to America including the Fair Isle sweater, knitted vests, "plus fours," the Scottish gillie shoe, and the Windsor knot. Unlike his father, George V, he preferred more informal comfortable clothing, as did many other young men of the period. The new leisure and sports clothing of the 1920s was a reflection of this trend.

UNDERGARMENTS

The popular one-piece "union suit," also called "long johns," was a combination of an undershirt and underpants. In winter they were made of knitted wool with long sleeves and legs, a buttoned fly, and a "drop seat" for convenience. Light-weight cotton dimity B.V.D.s were worn in summer. They were sleeveless with a U-neck and loose knee-length legs. Separate undershirts and underpants were also available.

After the demise of the ankle boot, socks became more visible and as a result more decorative. Patterned socks were worn in soft combinations of blue, brown, tan, and gray. They could be purchased in cotton, silk, rayon, or wool.

Many socks were embroidered over the ankles with vertical arrows, called "clocks." This fashion has waxed and waned ever since its introduction in the 16th century.

Adjustable hose garters were worn to support the socks. They were made of leather and striped elastic webbing, with one or two metal garters.

Ribbed knee-length knicker socks featured decorative plaid, Argyle, and geometric turnovers.

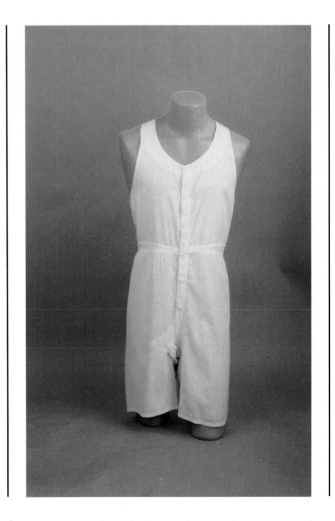

Summer union suit of pin check nainsook, cotton-knit waist insert, buttoned flap seat.

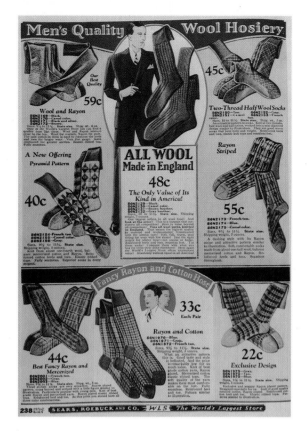

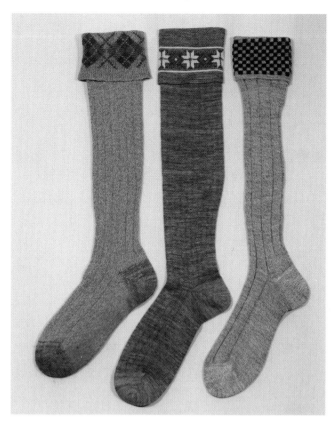

Men's wool, rayon and cotton socks in grid and geometric patterns. Sears, Roebuck and Co., 1928-29.

Brown and blue gray wool knee socks with argyle and other geometric patterned cuffs.

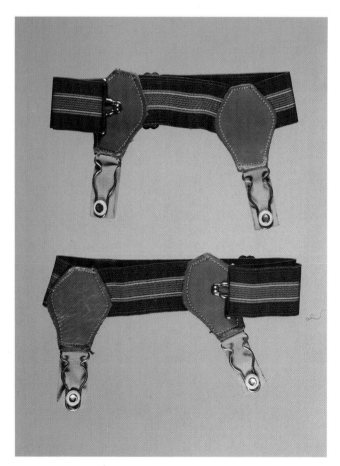

Elastic hose garters with leather tabs.

SLEEPWEAR AND LOUNGEWEAR

There were two styles of sleepwear worn by men during the 1920s. First, were the ankle-length flannel nightshirts, a holdover from the Victorian era. Second, were the flannel or broadcloth pajamas, offered in both cardigan and pullover styles. The most common fastenings for men's nightwear were decorative Chinese frogs.

When Noel Coward appeared on stage in a "dressing gown" in 1924, he set a new style in loungewear for men. Dressing gowns were a longer version of the smoking jacket and were made of wool, camel hair, cashmere, or *vicuña*. They featured a tasseled cord at the waist.

Soft blanket cloth robes in plaids, stripes, and geometric prints were popular for both sexes and all ages, throughout the decade. They were made in the shawl or notched collar styles and featured tasseled silk cord ties.

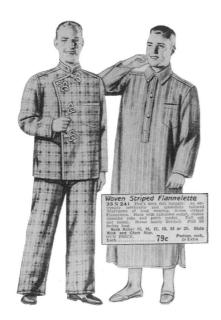

Men's flannelette nightwear—pajamas with frog closures and nightshirt. Charles William Stores, 1927-28.

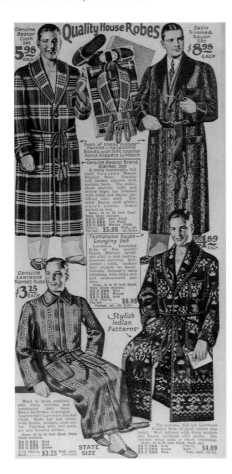

Three blanket robes with rayon tasseled girdles, one rayon robe with contrasting satin lapels, cuffs, and sash. Charles Williams Stores, 1927-28.

FORMAL WEAR

A gentlemen's full-dress suit consisted of a black or midnight blue worsted "swallow-tailed" coat (also called a "tailcoat" or "tails") with matching trousers. It featured satin or faille revers (lapels) and stripes along the pants seams.

A waist-length white piqué waistcoat (vest) was worn under the jacket. Vests were double or single-breasted and generally had a narrow collar. They were made with buttons or with button holes for studs. Backless vests were also available.

The starched white dress shirt had a bib front and detachable collar. A stiff "wing" collar was fastened to the shirt using collar buttons. Decorative studs were used to fasten the shirt front, while cuff links were used to fasten the French-style cuffs. (For more information on studs and cufflinks, refer to jewelry section at the end of this chapter.)

The proper neckwear for tails was a white bow tie. A shiny black silk "topper" (top hat), white kid gloves, patent leather oxfords or evening pumps, a white silk handkerchief for the breast pocket, and a *boutonnière* for the lapel completed the ensemble.

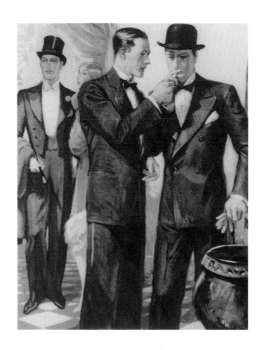

Top hat and tails. / Bowler with single and double-breasted tuxedos. Hart Schaffner & Marx Clothes, 1926.

165

SEMIFORMAL WEAR

The semiformal suit was called a tuxedo or "tux" by Americans, a "dinner jacket" by the English, and "*le smoking*" by the French. This comfortable alternative to tails was created, in 1886, by the affluent gentlemen of Tuxedo Park, New York. It was patterned after the smoking jacket and was designed to be worn for small dinner parties. Tuxedos were made of black or midnight blue worsted, with satin or faille lapels and trouser stripes. They were either single or double-breasted and featured a notched collar or peaked lapels. Some early single-breasted models were fastened in the front with a "link button," similar to a cuff link.

White waistcoats were single or double-breasted with narrow collars. Dress shirts had stiff, detachable wing collars and were fastened with studs. The tuxedo was always worn with a black bow tie. (When the words "black tie" appeared on an invitation it informed the guests that a tuxedo was required.) A bowler was the proper hat style to wear with the tuxedo. The remaining accessories were essentially the same as those worn with tails.

According to *Esquire's Encyclopedia of 20th Century Men's Fashion,* younger men favored more informal comfortable clothing such as dress shirts with soft attached collars and double-breasted dinner jackets which did not require a waistcoat.

SUITS

CONSERVATIVE SUIT

1920-1923

The conservative man's suit had a fitted jacket, a high slightly nipped-in waist, and narrow rounded shoulders. Notched collars and peaked lapels were high, short, and narrow. Both single and double-breasted jackets were available in two and three button versions. Some early models were fastened in front with a link button, others retained an attached belt, a carry-over from the teens.

Jazz suits with nipped-in waists and narrow trousers, late teens-early twenties. Hart, Schaffner and Marx.

Suits usually came with five-button vests. Since the trousers normally wore out before the jacket, many suits were offered with a pair and a spare. Popular colors for suits were black, gray, tan, brown, and navy. Typical suit fabrics were worsted, mohair, cashmere, herringbone, tweed, and Palm Beach cloth.

1924-1930

Suits during the last half of the decade were longer and roomier. Jackets featured broader shoulders and straighter lines with a less defined waist in its natural position. Trousers were also fuller with pleats at the waist.

Brooks Brothers was known for its well-tailored classic suits for the conservative male.

JAZZ SUIT

The jazz suit was a popular fad for young men, circa 1919-1923. It consisted of a tight-fitting jacket with a high nipped-in waist (remarkably similar to the women's high-waisted silhouette of the period). Trousers were short and very slender with narrow cuffs just over the ankles. These suits had a rather skimpy look about them, as though they were made for a smaller person.

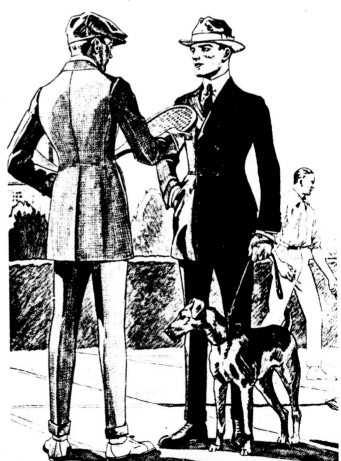

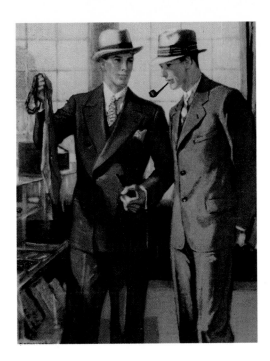

Double-breasted suit with homburg. / Single-breasted suit with snap brim hat. Hart Schaffner & Marx, 1926.

TROUSERS

Cuffs were added to the hems of mens' trousers circa the turn of the century. Front creases were adopted by young men after the First World War. Trousers were made with button flies until the early 1930s, when they were replaced by zippers. Wool flannel became a popular fabric for trousers during the twenties.

There was a major change in the fit of young men's trousers from 1920 to 1929, as the width of the legs passed from one extreme to the other. In the late teens and early 20s, pants were extremely snug, with cuffs ending just above the ankles. This created a skimpy, inadequate appearance.

In 1925, however, the undergraduates at Oxford University, began wearing trousers with wide baggy legs. These pants measured 25-30 inches around the knee, thus the name "Oxford bags." Legend has it that the Oxford rowing team wore the wide-leg pants over their knickers, which were unacceptable attire for classes. They became a popular fad for American college men during the late 20s and early 30s.

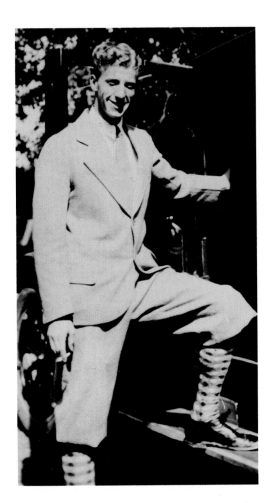

Author's father-in-law William Laubner wearing a knicker suit with wide lapels and patterned knicker socks.

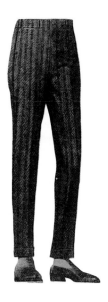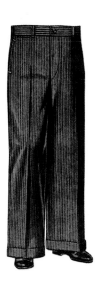

Compare the short tight trousers worn by young men in 1920 (Montgomery Ward), with the longer fuller "Oxford bags" style trousers of 1930 (National Bellas Hess).

SHIRTS AND COLLARS

A majority of the dress shirts offered in the early 1920s were collarless with a narrow band at the neck. The band had two button holes (front and back) which corresponded to holes in the detachable shirt collars. Collars were secured to the shirt by means of two collar buttons.

Stiff, semi stiff, and soft white detachable shirt collars were made in round, pointed, and wing-collar styles. Fabric collars which could be washed and starched were called "laundered" collars. Stiff celluloid collars were advertised as "cleanable" since they could be easily wiped with a damp cloth. (Men stored their collars in collar boxes or "bandboxes" covered with genuine or imitation leather.) More comfortable shirts with attached collars were also offered and began to replace collarless shirts by the end of the decade.

Dress shirts were made of percale, broadcloth, madras, khaki, oxford cloth, tissue silk, and mercerized cotton. They were made in stripes, solids, and mini prints.

Arrow, Van Heusen, and Manhattan were three of the well-known shirt manufacturers of the decade.

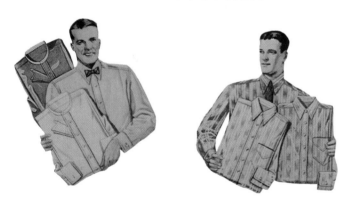

Dress shirts with and with out collars. Charles Williams Stores, 1927-28.

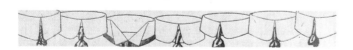

Men's shirt collars including one formal wing collar. Montgomery Ward, 1920-21.

NECKWEAR

Suit jackets, vests, and sweaters of the early 1920s had high-neck openings which obscured all but the tops of ties. For this reason many of the early ties were short, ending three to four-inches above the waist. Colorful knitted four-in-hand ties were popular throughout the decade. They were made of silk or rayon in colorful stripes with square cut ends.

Woven neckties were made of silk or rayon, in foulard, jacquard, moiré, and crepe de chine. Black, maroon, blue, purple, brown, green, and gray were the favorite colors.

During the early 1920s, "bat wing" bow ties were offered with horseshoe-shaped ends. The 1929 Sears, Roebuck and Co. catalog offered a new "butterfly" bow tie with thistle-shaped ends. "Made-up" bow and four-in-hand ties were also available throughout the period.

In 1926, Jeanne Lanvin became the first designer to open a men's division featuring men's accessories.

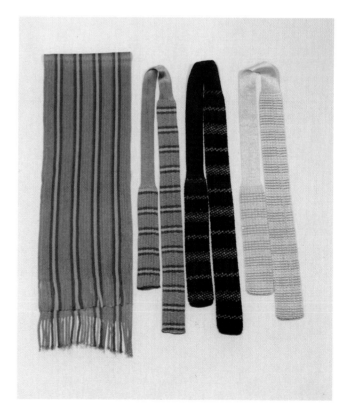

Rayon knitted muffler and four-in-hand knitted ties. *Courtesy of William R. Fryer.*

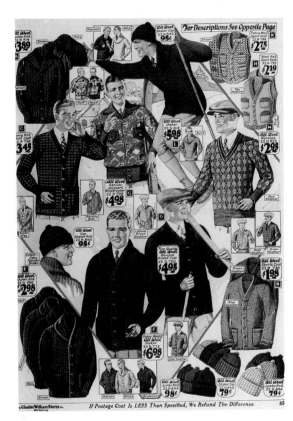

Wool cap, varsity letter sweater, "plus fours" with button fly, and knicker socks.

Men's sweaters—(A, E, F, L) Shaker knit; (K, H) wool knit sport vests; (B, C, D) V-neck cardigans; (G) lumberjack jacket; (M) Fair Isle or cricket sweater. Charles William, 1927-28.

SPORTSWEAR

INFORMAL LEISURE-TIME CLOTHING

Knicker Suit

The knicker suit was worn for leisure activities and consisted of a sport jacket and matching knickers. They were generally made of corduroy, linen, herringbone, or tweed.

Sweaters

"Fair Isle" sweaters were made in geometric stripes and the popular Argyle pattern. They were worn tucked in or out of the trousers. They were also referred to as "cricket" sweaters in mail-order catalogs of the period.

Heavy shaker-knit cardigan and pullover sweaters with high shawl collars were often worn in place of a jacket.

ACTIVE SPORTS CLOTHING

Bathing

Purple wool bathing suit (back view featuring cutouts). *Courtesy of Thomas H. Weaber.* / Black wool suit (same style - front view). *Courtesy of Sue Steiner.* / Straw boater.

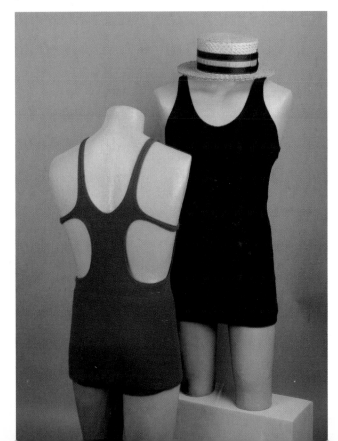

By 1920, the two-piece woolen bathing suit had been replaced by the new California-style one-piece suit. This style consisted of a wool tank top with short matching trunks attached at the waist. During the latter half of the decade, these suits acquired large openings which extended from under the arm to the center of the back. Common colors were red, purple, yellow, pale blue, or the combination of black and orange.

Golf

The patterned "Fair Isle" pullover sweater was popularized by the Prince of Wales, when he wore it to tee off at St. Andrews in 1922. It was worn with "plus fours," a term used by the British Army to describe the baggy knickers which were worn four-inches below the knee. Plus fours were introduced by the Prince of Wales during his visit to America in 1924. A golf cap and knicker socks completed the golfer's attire.

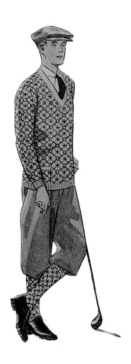

Golf ensemble including cap, Fair Isle sweater, "plus-fours," and knicker socks. *Town & Country*, 4/26. *Courtesy of Judy Carpenter.*

Tennis

The standard men's tennis outfit included a long-sleeved white shirt (with the sleeves rolled up to the elbows) and white flannel trousers.

The United States tennis champion Bill Tilden started a vogue for the white or cream-colored cable knit tennis sweater which featured a contrasting stripe at the V-neck, cuffs, and waistband. This classic style was also worn by English cricket players.

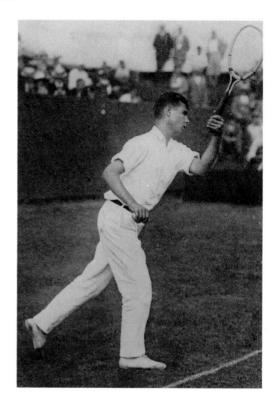

John Doeg of California wearing typical tennis outfit—white shirt, pants, and athletic shoes. *Vogue*, 9/15/26.

Skiing

Heavy coat sweaters, patterned Fair Isle sweaters, or waterproof jackets were worn with trousers or knickers. A knitted cap, a muffler (scarf), and gloves completed the outfit.

Horseback Riding

American horsemen looked to the English for the style and cut of riding habits. For ordinary riding, a tweed "hacking" jacket was worn in dark brown, gray, tan, or black. Jodhpurs were usually gray, fawn, or tan. A riding shirt, a tie or stock, a bowler or soft felt hat, and black or brown riding boots completed the outfit. (See the photo of a man's riding habit in Chapter 6.)

OUTERWEAR

ULSTER

The high-waisted silhouette of the late teens and early twenties was noticeable in men's overcoats (top coats) as well as suits. The double-breasted Ulster was named after the province in Ireland where it was first introduced in the 1860s. It was made of heavy wool with a wide-notched or fur-trimmed shawl collar and featured a full belt or belted back only. The "zero weather" Ulster was lined with fur. Ulsters of the later years had straight lines with no defined waist.

CHESTERFIELD

The Chesterfield coat was introduced in the 1840s by the fashionable Earl of Chesterfield. The most recognizable feature of this formal coat was the black velvet collar. Chesterfields were usually single-breasted with a fly front which concealed the buttons, however, double-breasted versions did exist.

TRENCHCOAT

The trenchcoat was first worn by British officers during the First World War. It was adopted as an all-purpose coat for civilian use in the 1920s, and has been a classic favorite ever since. It was commonly made of beige waterproof gabardine.

RACCOON COAT

The coat most associated with the 1920s was the raccoon coat. This large bulky fur coat was a favorite among college men and women for football games and rides in open roadsters. (For a photograph and description, refer to Chapter 7.)

MACKINAW JACKET

The double-breasted Mackinaw jacket originated in Mackinaw City, Michigan, in 1811. This heavy wool plaid jacket featured a shawl collar and a self belt.

LUMBERJACK JACKET

The wool plaid "lumberjack" jacket featured a convertible collar with knitted cuffs and banded waist.

HAIR AND HATS

Young men rejected the short military-style hair cut associated with the war years. They preferred slightly longer hair which they parted in the center or just slightly off center. It was plastered down with pomade, giving it a slick shiny appearance called "patent leather" hair.

Many of the hats worn by men during the 1920s were introduced in the 19th century. Men were slowly abandoning the more formal styles in favor of more casual hats.

Adams and Stetson were two of the major companies manufacturing these hats in the 1920s.

TOP HAT

The most formal of all hats was the top hat made of shiny silk or beaver. It was introduced in the early 19th century, and was worn as a businessman's hat for day or evening. By the 1920s, this hat was reserved for formal dress with tails. (See formal wear photo.)

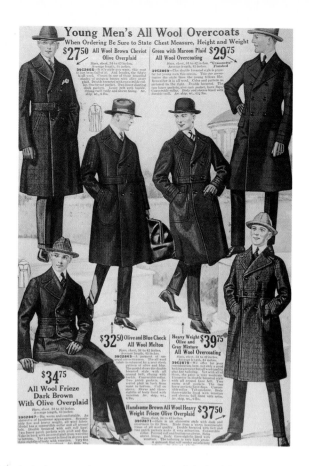

Men's high-waisted overcoats with self belt. Montgomery Ward, 1920-21.

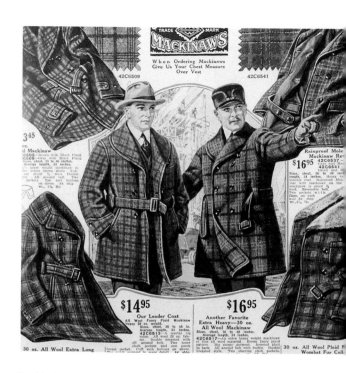

Double-breasted wool plaid mackinaws. Montgomery Ward, 1920/21.

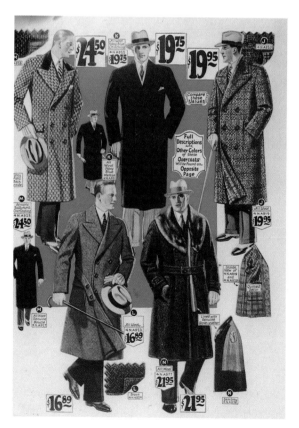

Men's overcoats including a double-breasted adaptation of chesterfield and beaver trimmed ulster. Note: homburgs and snap-brim hats. Charles William Stores, 1927-28.

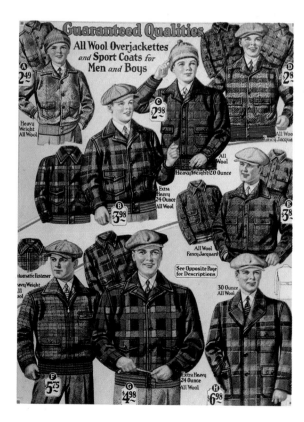

Wool plaid lumberjack "overjackettes" with banded waist. M.W. Savage Co., 1927/28.

BOWLER

The bowler was introduced in the 1850s by a London businessman. It was made of hard black or brown felt with a dome-shaped crown and a narrow brim which curled up at the sides. It was worn for semiformal dress with a tuxedo and by middle-class businessmen in the city. It was also worn as part of the riding habit and by spectators at horse races, thus the American name "derby." (See formal wear photo.)

HOMBURG

The Homburg was popularized in the 1870s by the future King Edward VII after a visit to the spa and resort town of Homburg, Germany. Appropriate for day or evening wear, it had a stiff felt crown with a long crease which ran from front to back.

FEDORA

The fedora was introduced in 1882. It featured a crease which ran over the top of the crown (front to back) similar to the Homburg, but was made of soft felt. Dandies preferred to wear this hat with the brim turned down on one side, and up on the other. In the mid twenties, college men turned the front of the brim down. It was then referred to as a "snap brim" or a "swagger hat."

TELESCOPE

The telescope or "pork-pie" sport hat had a crease around the edge of the flat crown. The brim was worn down in front and up in back.

BOATER

The straw boater was originally worn for punting on the Thames River in England. When the Prince of Wales (later Edward the VII) donned the boater in 1896, it became an immediate success. It was worn as a sport hat in America from June through September until 1930.

PANAMA HAT

Panama hats were made in Ecuador of light-weight South American reed. They were made with a ridged crown and were unlined which made them a cool choice for summer.

CAP

Caps were worn by working-class men for everyday or by the well-to-do for sport. They were made of nubby tweeds, plaids, checks, herringbones, corduroy, and poplin in brown, gray, and navy.

COLLEGE DINK

College freshman were required to wear a small cap, called a dink, which was made of felt in the school's colors. It was worn during "hazing" (usually the first two or three weeks of school). Upperclassmen could easily recognize the lowly freshman and give them small tasks to do as an initiation. Shedding the dink at the end of hazing became a much anticipated right of passage.

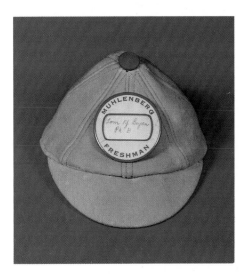

Felt dink—type worn by freshmen during hazing at Muhlenberg College, Allentown, Pennsylvania. *Courtesy of Tom Y. Bryan.*

BILLFOLDS

During the 20s, paper currency measured 7 7/16" X 3 1/8." It was reduced to the current size (6 1/8 x 2 5/8) during July of 1929. Wallets had to be larger to accommodate these big bills and were often folded in thirds to form a less cumbersome tri-fold billfold. Common materials were calf skin, ostrich, steerhide, and pig skin. They were also available with decorative hand-tooled designs.

SHOES

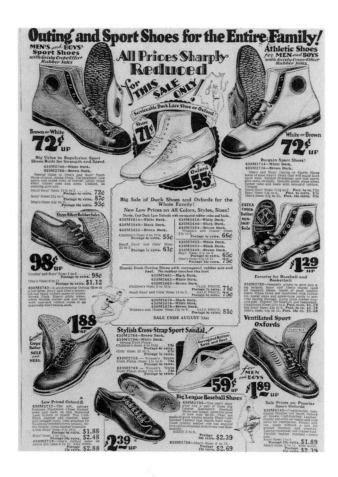

Mens' and boys' athletic shoes for tennis, basketball, running, and baseball, *Bellas Hess & Company*, 1928. *Courtesy of Suzanjoy M. Checksfield.*

GILLIE

On his visit to America, the Prince of Wales introduced the gillie, a shoe worn with a kilt by Scottish dancers. This tongueless shoe was laced through leather loops, instead of eyelets.

OXFORD

The oxford had all but replaced the lace-up boot in popularity. The growing interest in sports led to a need for sport oxfords with crepe-rubber soles. Toes were slowly evolving from semi-round during the early twenties to square towards the end of the decade. Black, brown, tan, and white were the predominant colors. Many styles were decorated with broguings (small perforations).

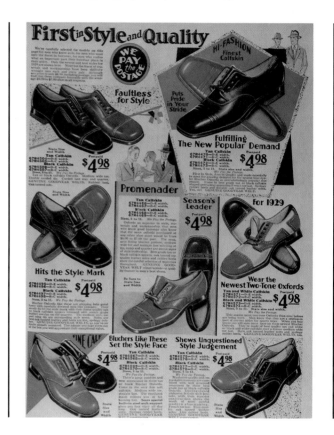

Men's square toe shoes including two-toned Oxfords (forerunner of the spectator). Sears, Roebuck and Co., 1928-29.

SPECTATOR

Two-toned oxfords were made of white buckskin with black or brown leather toes, insteps, and quarters (back). Broguings were often placed along the edges of the dark leather. These sport shoes were later called spectators ("co-respondents" in the U.K.).

SADDLE SHOE

White buckskin oxfords with brown or black saddles were popular for sport and were often made with rubber soles. They were referred to as saddle shoes by the mid-thirties.

JEWELRY

RINGS

There were many types of rings worn by men during the 1920s. The belcher setting (popular from the 1870s through the 1920s), was characterized by six heavy prongs or claws which reached up to held the stone in place. Also in vogue were signet, cameo, emblem, and solitaire rings with a variety of stones. Black onyx rings with diamond or initial centers were also a favorite.

DRESS SETS

Dress sets were designed for those special occasions when a dress shirt was required. These sets contained fancy studs and matching cuff links. Dress shirts were made with buttonholes on either side of the center-front opening. Studs (removable buttons) were slipped through the corresponding buttonholes fastening the two sides of the shirt together.

Each dress-shirt sleeve contained a "French cuff" featuring buttonholes on either side of the placket. A cuff link was inserted through each pair of holes, thus fastening the cuff. Cuff links were produced in many styles and shapes. The "loose link" or "cuff button" style contained two parts resembling buttons which were connected by a metal link. In the late 1920s and 1930s, the "snap cuff" or "separable cuff link" became popular. This style contained two parts which snapped together. They were also known by such trade names as "Kum-a-part," "Stalokt," "Pressit," and "Du-Lock."

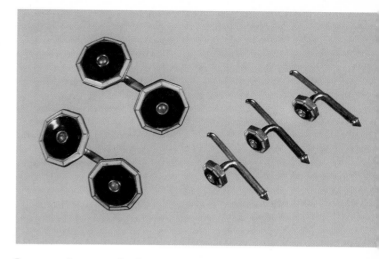

Five-piece dress set with white enameled rims, black glass disks with half pearls centers. Contains two octagonal loose link cuff links and three matching shirt studs (with sliding bars). Marked: Rolled Gold Plate. *Courtesy of William Laubner, Sr.*

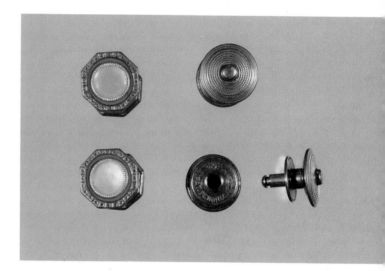

Two pair of snap-style cuff links. / Engraved nickel rim, green celluloid border, mother-of-pearl center. Marked: SNAP LINK. / Gold-filled cuff links with engine-turnings. Marked: TISCO LOCK, Pat. Pend.

Nine-piece gold-filled smoked mother of pearl dress set in original presentation box. Contains two loose link cuff links, three shirt studs (with sliding bars), and four vest studs with removable cotter pins. Marked: Gold-filled. *Courtesy of William Laubner, Sr.*

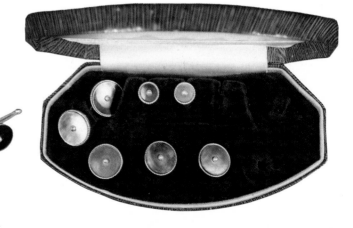

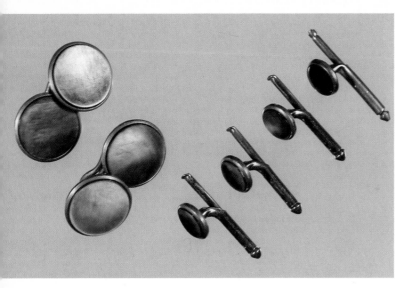

Six-piece chrome-plated dress set containing two mother-of-pearl loose link cuff links and four matching shirt studs (with sliding bars). *Courtesy of William Laubner, Sr.*

Common shapes for studs and cuff links were the circle, octagon, hexagon, barrel, oval, and modified square and rectangle. They were made of platinum; 10K, 12K, and 14K solid gold; rolled gold plate; gold filled; and sterling silver. These items could be engine-turned, chased, brocaded, embossed, hammered, inlaid, enameled, or hand engraved with the wearer's initials. They were decorated with anything from diamonds and sapphires to jade, mother-of-pearl, amethyst, and carnelian.

SCARF AND COLLAR PINS

Scarf pins (also known as stickpins or tie pins) were used to fasten four-in-hand ties or ascots to the shirt. The decorative end usually contained one or more stones placed in a geometric white gold setting. A clutch or guard was placed on the opposite end to secure the pin to the tie. Growing in popularity were collar pins, which were fastened to each side of the new soft collars to hold them in the "proper position." Short clothespin-style tie clips were also gaining favor.

WATCHES AND WATCH CHAINS

A man generally wore his pocket watch in a vest pocket, anchoring it with a watch chain which was fastened to one of the buttonholes. On hot summer days, however, men shed their vests, creating a need for an alternative safety device for watches. One such device was a short chain with a button on the opposite end. When the watch was placed in the breast pocket, the short attached chain was fastened to the lapel by pushing the decorative button through the buttonhole (from the reverse side).

For the gentleman who wished to place his watch in the fob pocket of his trousers, a short watch chain was used with a "belt slide" on the opposite end. The metal slide was slipped over the belt to a position over the fob pocket. Watch slides were often produced in sets containing a matching belt buckle.

The wristwatch grew in popularity during the 1920s, eventually replacing the pocket watch.

Monogramming was extremely popular in the twenties. Small rectangular *cartouches* were created for this purpose on jewelry, belt buckles, belt slides, watches, cigarette and cigar cases, lighters, and flasks. (See Chapter 9 for typical monograms.)

It was also popular to adorn men's jewelry with emblems of the fraternal orders such as the Elks, the Masons, the Knights of Columbus, the Odd Fellows, and the Shriners.

White gold scarf pin (stick pin), one square set diamond, four triangular sapphires, safety clutch on shaft. *Courtesy of William Laubner, Sr.*

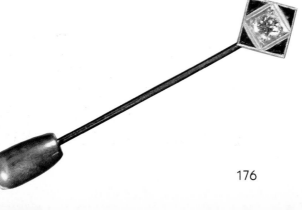

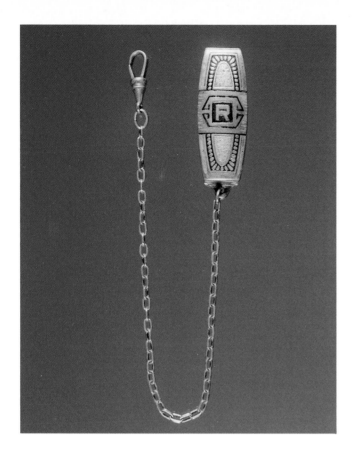

Silver-plated brass belt sleeve with watch chain and hook, engraved initial "R". Marked: Kichok Beltogram, Kickok Plate.

Gold-plated lapel watch chain with engraved button and watch hook. Marked: D. CO, c. early 1920s.

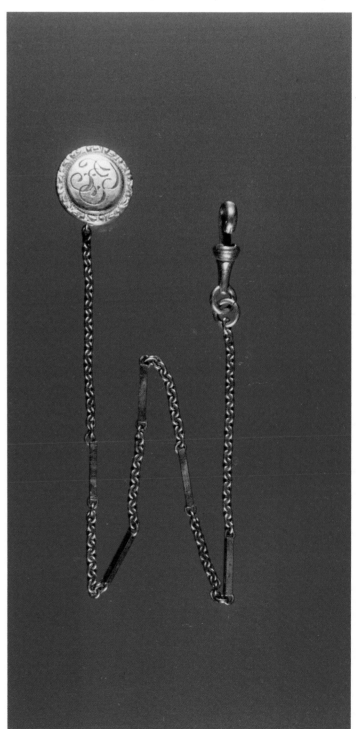

Man wearing a watch in his lapel pocket with the watch chain attached to the buttonhole of his lapel.

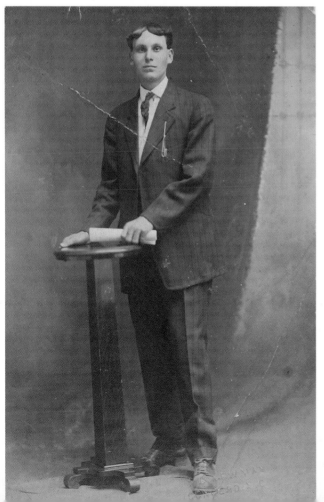

177

CHAPTER 14
UNIFORMS

DOMESTIC SERVANTS

During this prosperous period, it was customary for wealthy families to hire domestic servants to perform the day to day household duties. This was so common, in fact, that garment manufacturers advertised servants' uniforms in women's magazines of the period. Just as the lady of the house had certain types of clothing for certain times of the day, so too did her servants. In general, afternoon and evening uniforms were more formal in appearance than morning uniforms.

MAID

The maid's afternoon uniform consisted of a taffeta, crepe, moiré, or poplin dress in dark blue, green, brown, burgundy, or plum. Gray or black was preferred by the older, more "conservative houses" or for evening affairs. The waistline for maids' uniforms remained primarily in its natural position. Matching white collar, cuffs, apron, and gathered or pleated headpiece were standard. The headpiece was worn over the area between the crown of the head and the forehead. It was tied in the back with an attached ribbon. For fancy afternoon or evening wear, these items might be made of lace.

Waitress uniforms of the period followed the same basic lines as the maid's.

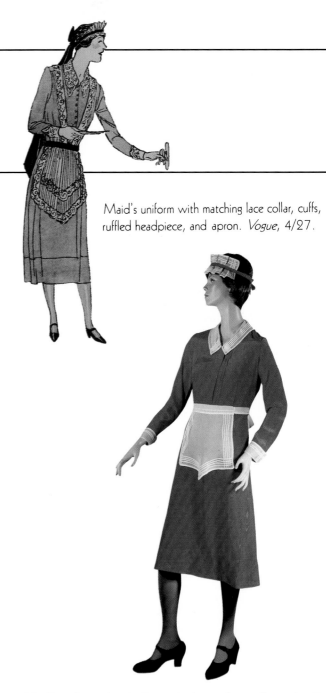

Maid's uniform with matching lace collar, cuffs, ruffled headpiece, and apron. *Vogue*, 4/27.

Maid's uniform of red silk moiré, sheer white collar and cuffs with ribbon trim. (Headpiece and apron recreated using period photographs.) *Courtesy of Cedar Crest College, gift of Sue Steiner.*

BUTLER

For afternoon, the well-dressed butler wore a black tail coat and matching vest, striped trousers, and a black for-in-hand or bow tie. For evening, a black tail coat with matching vest and trousers, and a black or white bow tie were proper.

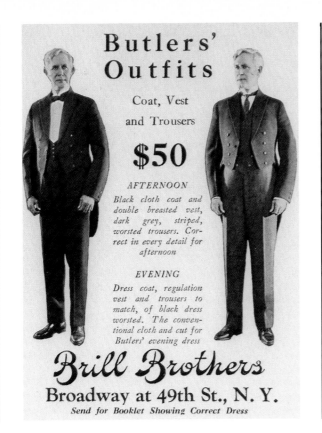
Butler's uniforms. / Evening - black worsted tail coat, trousers, and matching single-breasted vest; black bow tie. / Afternoon - black worsted tail coat and double-breasted vest, gray striped trousers, four-in-hand necktie. *Vogue*, 10/25.

CHAUFFEUR

The chauffeur's ensemble included a peaked cap with matching single or double-breasted jacket and trousers. Jodhpur-style pants and knee-high leather boots were optional. For colder weather, a double-breasted "great coat" (overcoat) was worn.

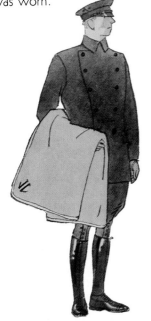
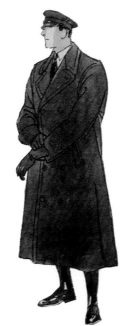

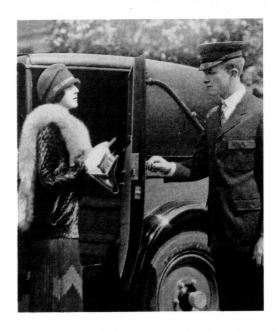

Chauffeur's uniform—peaked cap, jacket with high notched collar and three "bellows" pockets, trousers. Note: fur piece. *Town & Country*, 9/26. *Courtesy of Judy Carpenter.*

GOVERNESS

Nursemaids or "nannies" wore *cloche*-style hats and capes for walks in the park with their *charges*.

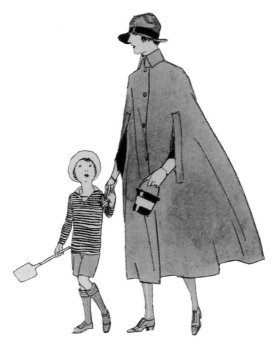

Governess' attire—vagabond hat and cape. *Vogue*, 4/27.

Chauffeur's uniforms. / Peaked cap, jacket with high collar, *jodhpurs*, and boots (since there were no heaters in cars until the 1930s, a car robe or blanket was handy to take along in cold weather). / Overcoat with notched collar, gloves, and boots. *Vogue*, 4/27.

179

COOK

Uniforms for cooks were traditionally made of white cotton. A white cotton cap was worn to keep loose hair from falling into the food.

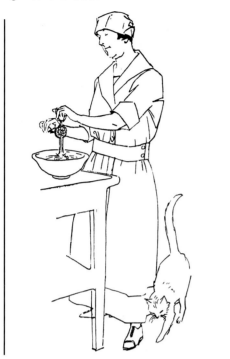

Cook's uniform and watching cap. *Vogue, 4/27.*

Dietitian's muslin uniform including white studs, teens-1922. *Courtesy of Cedar Crest Alumnae Museum, gift of Gerry Coraor.*

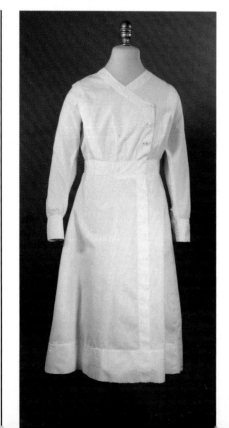

HOTEL, BOUTIQUE, AND DEPARTMENT STORE EMPLOYEES

DOORMAN

It was customary for posh hotels and department stores to station a doorman at the entrance. It was his duty to open doors and assist people to and from their cars. A doorman wore a large broad-shouldered overcoat with contrasting collar, cuffs, and pocket flaps. Braided trim and brass buttons were added for a touch of distinction.

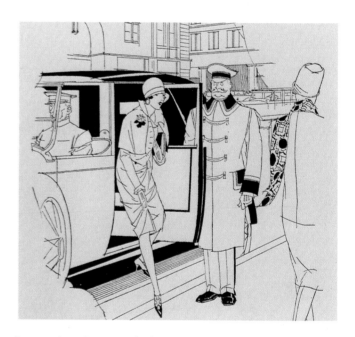

Doorman's uniform—peaked cap; broad-shouldered overcoat with contrasting collar, cuffs, and pocket flaps, braided trim. *Vogue, 6/26. Courtesy of Richard Groman.*

BELLBOY

Bellboys were employed at hotels to assist the guests with their luggage and packages. A bellboy's uniform consisted of a red pillbox hat with gold braid and chin strap, a red waist-length jacket with a stand-up collar, and black trousers. The jacket featured gold braid at the neck and cuffs, and a double row of brass buttons arranged in a large V.

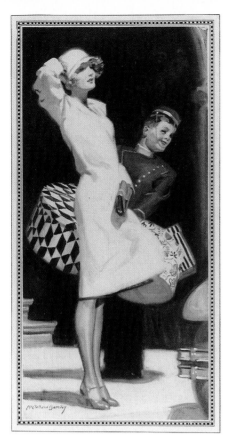

Bellhop's uniform—typical pillbox hat with gold trim and chin strap, waist-length coat with brass buttons. *Vogue*, 4/15/27.

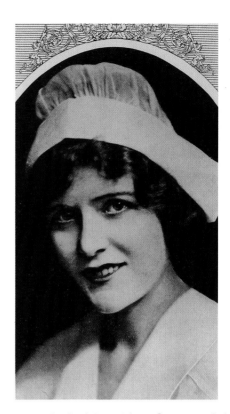

Nurse's cap pictured in Paul Jones Nurse Costumes ad. *Vogue*, 10/25.

HEALTH CARE WORKERS

NURSE

Nurses uniforms followed the prevailing silhouette and hem length of the period. They were usually white but striped seersucker was also common. Each nursing school had its own unique style of starched white cap worn by its graduates.

Nurse's uniform—dress with high waistband of the early 20s. L'Aiglon, 1922.

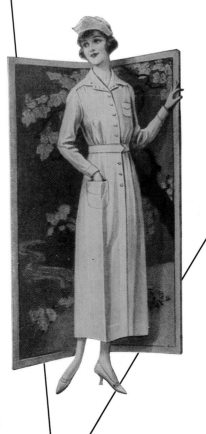

CHAPTER 15
CHILDREN'S WEAR

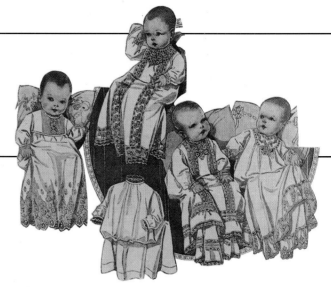

INFANT'S WEAR

Layettes were available for the newborn which included dresses, bonnets, nightgowns, sleeping bags, sacques, petticoats, kimonos, undershirts, bibs, towels, washcloths, booties, diapers, and blankets.

Both girl and boy babies were dressed in elaborate long white cotton lawn dresses trimmed with bows, ribbon rosettes, embroidery, pin tucks, shirring, and inserts of lace. They were often available with matching bonnets. Long white coats with attached capes were worn over these dresses in cooler weather.

Infant's cotton lawn dresses decorated with embroidery, tucks, lace, and ribbon rosettes. Montgomery Ward, 1920-21.

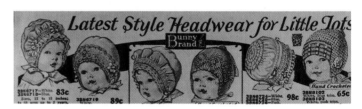

Baby bonnets. Sears, Roebuck and Co., 1928-29.

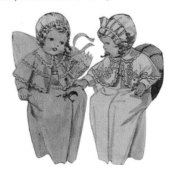

Cape coats with matching bonnets. / Bedford cord coat. / Cotton cashmere trimmed with silk embroidery. Montgomery Ward, 1920-21.

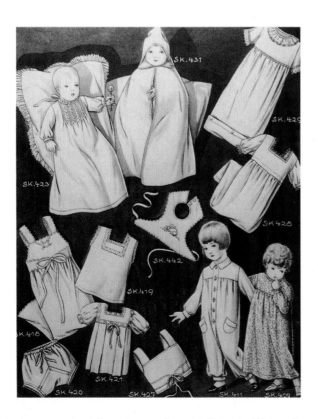

Baby layette and toddler nightwear *Reinach's Review of Fashion*, Paris, 1928. *Courtesy of Lehigh County Historical Society.*

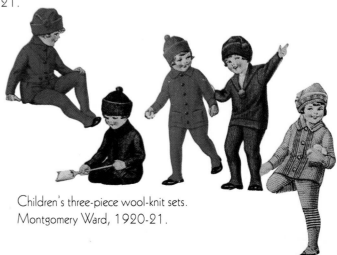

Children's three-piece wool-knit sets. Montgomery Ward, 1920-21.

GIRLS' WEAR AND ACCESSORIES

Little girls wore "bloomer dresses" which were, as the name implies, loose sack-style dresses with matching panties, just barely visible below the skirt hem. Embroidery, smocking, ribbons, and ribbon rosettes were popular forms of decoration.

Matching big-and-little-sister frocks by Hollander were featured in the April 1927 issue of *Vogue* magazine. These simple styles were designed for girls between the ages of two and twelve.

Young girls wore miniature wedding dresses with flowered headpieces and veils for their First Communion.

In winter, coats with fur collars and leggings with new slide fasteners (zippers) were popular for girls. Three-piece knitted sets consisting of a hat, a sweater, and leggings were also common.

For special occasions, girls wore poke bonnets or mini versions of the *cloches* worn by their mothers. Headbands for young girls were often decorated with ribbon flowers to complement a particular party dress.

Miniature ring and armor-mesh bags were all the rage. Some of these bags were just large enough to hold two or three coins.

Shoes for girls ranged from winter "hi-cut" boots to fancy patent leather strap shoes.

A popular gift for preteen girls was the celluloid brisé fan. It consisted of 20-24 individual pierced sticks, which were held together by a single strip of pastel ribbon. Dainty painted flowers were added for a feminine touch.

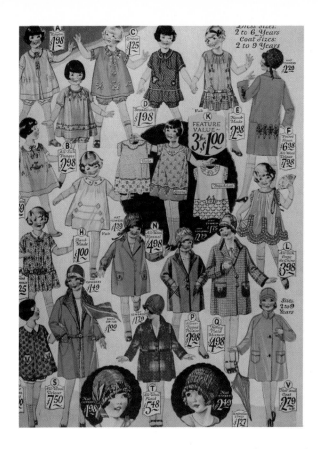

Little girls' bloomer dresses, coats, and hats. National Cloak and Suit Co., 1927.

Children's clothing - boys' two-piece suits, girls' bloomer and pre-teen dresses. *Delineator*, 6/23.

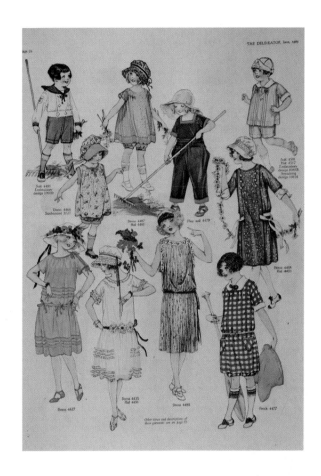

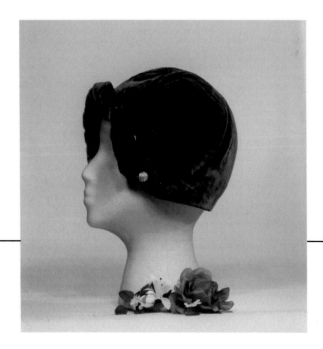

Ribbon bows and *bandeaux* for little girls. *Ribbon Art Book*, 1923.

French designer Jeanne Lanvin began her career making clothing for her young daughter, Marie-Blanche. Her attractive creations were much admired and she was soon designing outfits for the daughters of her friends. She is also known for her matching "mother-and-daughter dresses." Lanvin's trade mark, which appears on her labels and perfume bottles, was designed for her by the prominent fashion illustrator Paul Iribe. This logo contains a stylized illustration of a mother and daughter holding hands, a symbol of the close bond which she shared with her daughter.

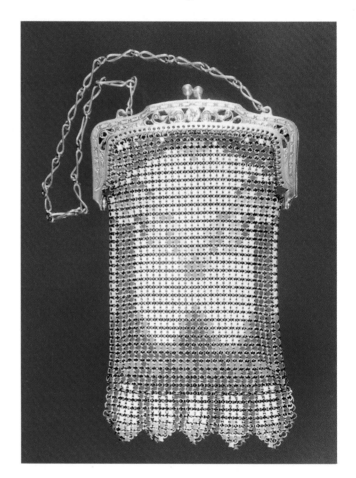

Child's enameled armor-mesh bag (3" x 5"), silver-plated openwork frame. Marked: Whiting & Davis. *Courtesy of Doris Caddock.*

Deep red silk velvet *cloche* with shirred brim, accented with rhinestone bottoms.

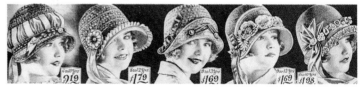

Girls' cloches. National Cloak & Suit Co., 1927.

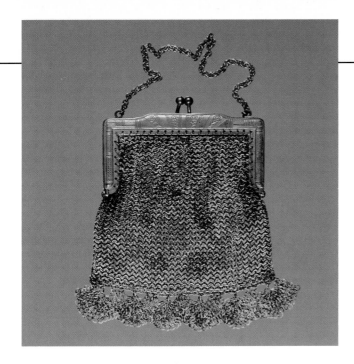

Child's small enameled ring-mesh bag (2 1/2" x 3 1/4") with gold-plated and enameled frame. Carried to Sunday School, c. 1929. *Courtesy of Cedar Crest Alumnae Museum, gift of Althea H. Mantz.*

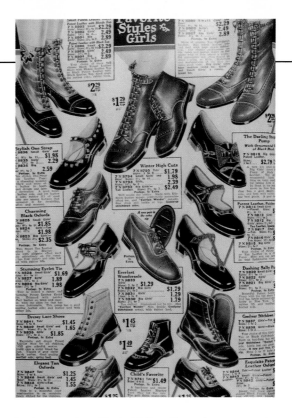

Girls' shoe styles, Charles William Store, Inc., 1927-28.

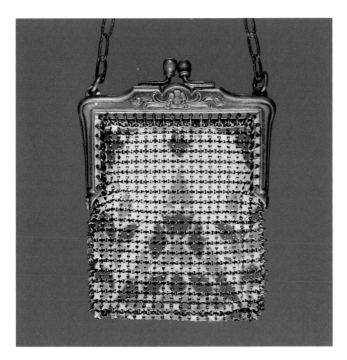

Child's enameled armor-mesh bag (2 1/4" x 3"), embossed silver-plated brass frame. *Courtesy of Nancy Blankowitsch.*

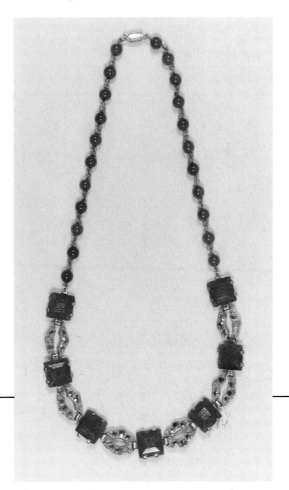

Girl's necklace made of synthetic lapis and base metal segments with artificial marcasite (silvered jet).

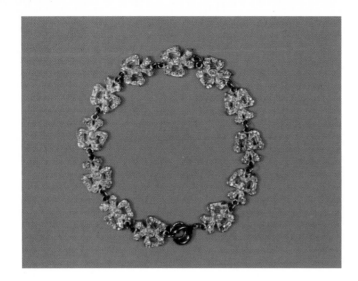

Bracelet made of tiny base metal bows decorated with rhinestones.

Sailor-style coats with matching hats were popular out-erwear for winter. Also popular were Ulster coats, which often featured a fur collar.

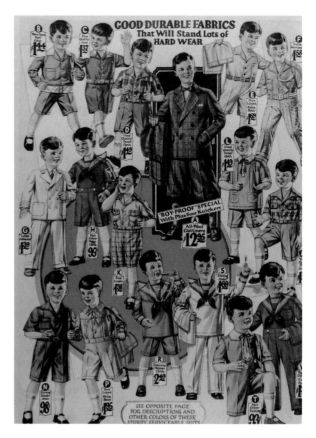

Boys' two-piece suits, knicker suit, and sailor suits. National Cloak and Suit Co. 1927.

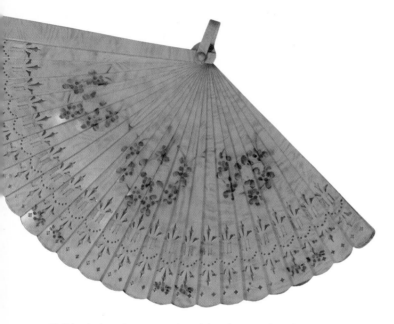

Celluloid *brisé* fan, pierced and hand painted with forget-me-nots, laced with pale blue satin ribbon.

Boys' white cotton two-piece suit, pants are buttoned to shirt, 1922. *Courtesy of Edward Mayer.*

BOYS' WEAR

Boys, one to four years old, wore suits consisting of a shirt with buttons at the waist with which to attach the short matching pants. Sailor versions of these suits were very popular. The "romper," worn by both sexes, was a one-piece combination of shirt and pants with elastic at the bottom of each leg.

During the early 20s, boys five to ten years old wore knicker suits with a belted jacket. These suits were a last vestige of the "Norfolk suit" which was popular at the turn of the century. The belt began to disappear from suits in the latter half of the decade. Suits for older boys often contained both long pants (for dress-up) and knickers (for sport).

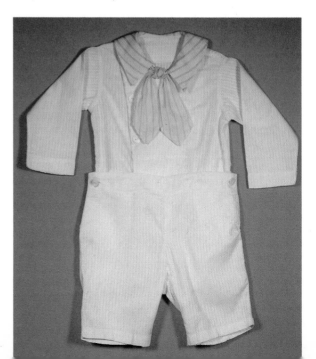

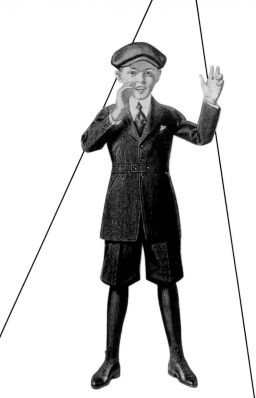

Boys' wool Norfolk-style knicker suit, wool cap, knicker socks, and "hi-cut" shoes. Montgomery Ward, 1920-21.

First Communion photo. Big girls—wearing white dresses with low belts, floral wreath headpieces with veils. / Little girl—bloomer dress. / Boys—Norfolk-style knicker suits, c. early 1920s.

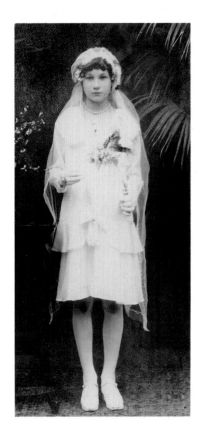

First Communion dress with dropped waist and layered skirt, floral decorated cap and veil, c.1925-30.

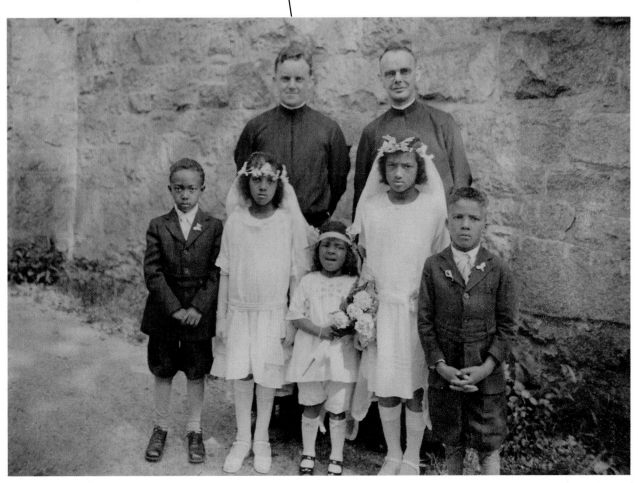

GLOSSARY
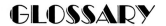

Capital letter = Long vowel sound
A = say   O = toe
E = see   U = true
I = tie   OO = food

Lower case letter = Short vowel sound
a = hat   o = lot
e = net   u = but
i = pig   oo = cook

There are some French words on this list which have become commonplace in the English language. They were often given an English pronunciation, however. In these cases I have listed both the French and the English pronunciations.

Agnès (ah-nyes)
French milliner who specialized in tailored sporty hats. She is remembered for her use of Cubist-style fabrics designed by such renowned artists as Piet Mondrian and Sonia Delaunay.

aigrette (A-gret)
Long straight white feathers from the egret (a member of the heron family). They were attached to the inside of the bandeau and worn over the center of the forehead as part of the evening ensemble.

Alençon lace (a-lon-sOn)
This needlepoint lace was originally made in Alençon, France, in the early 17th century. Floral designs were created on a fine net ground and outlined with heavy thread called *cordonnet* (cor-dO-nA).

androgynous
Bearing both male and female qualities, as the flat chested flappers who resembled boys. Origin: Greek—*andros* "man," and *gynacea* "woman."

anhk (ank)
A cross with a loop at the top, which is the ancient Egyptian symbol of eternal life. It is also called an "ansate cross."

appliqué (a-plE-kA)
A technique involving decorative pieces of fabric which are cut and either stitched or glued to another fabric. This technique can also be applied to leather for shoes and handbags. Origin: French—"applied to."

Argyle (ar-gIl)
A multicolored diamond pattern which was derived from the Scottish tartan of the Argyle clan. This classic geometric pattern became popular during the 1920s when it was used for woolen sweaters, socks, and scarves. Also spelled *Argyll* and *Argyl*.

Art Deco
A decorative art movement introduced to the world at the Parisian *Exposition International des Arts Décoratifs et Industriels Modernes* in 1925. Art Deco was characterized by geometric shapes, parallel lines, concentric circles, step patterns, sunbursts, waterfalls, fountains, stylized flowers (i.e. the Deco rose), and other abstract motifs.

Art Nouveau (art new-vO)
A decorative art movement (c. 1895-1915) characterized by fluid graceful lines, i.e. flowers with long swirling tendrils and women with long flowing hair. The width of these *wavy* lines also varied from thick to thin. Origin: French—*nouveau*—"new."

Arts and Crafts Movement
Introduced in the late 19th century, this movement promoted handmade decorative arts, as opposed to machine-made mass-produced items.

Assuit (ass-yout) stoles
Exotic linen mesh stoles imported from the ancient city of Assuit, Egypt. They were particularly popular after the discovery of King Tutankhamen's tomb in 1922. These rectangular stoles were decorated by hand with millions of shiny pieces of metal arranged in decorative patterns. After the introduction of Art Deco in 1925, many stoles were decorated with geometric patterns.

Astrakhan
1. In the late 19th century, this term referred to the curly fleece or pelt of the karakul lamb, raised in Astrakhan, USSR. It was also called Persian lamb. 2. Astrakhan cloth was a heavy knitted or woven fabric with a deep curly pile which was made to imitate Persian lamb.

Augustabernard
Born Augusta Bernard in Provence, France, she combined her two names when she opened her own shop in 1919. She designed clothing for the custom departments at Henri Bendel and Bergdorf Goodman. She is known for her simple timeless bias-cut crepe and satin evening gowns of the late 1920s through 1934 (when she retired).

avant-garde (a-von gard)
In a fashion context, this term is used to describe an unconventional new style. Origin: French—"leading part of an army."

Bakelite
The trade name for a synthetic resin or plastic named after its inventor, Belgian chemist L.H. Baekeland. It reached the height of popularity in the late 20s and 30s when it was molded or carved into colorful jewelry, buttons, and buckles. The most common colors were "catsup," "mustard," and "avocado."

Ballets Russe (ba-lA rOOs)
The Ballet Russe (French for Russian Ballet), directed by Serge Diaghilev, first performed in Paris in 1909. The vivid Middle Eastern costumes, designed by Léon Bakst, were the single most important influence on fashions of the teens. They inspired French couturier Paul Poiret who designed exotic oriental style garments and elegant turbans.

bandeau Fr. (bon-dO) pl. bandeaux (bon-dO) / Eng. (ban-dO)
1. A headband worn around the forehead. 2. An undergarment formed from a flat piece of fabric (without cups). It was fastened tightly over the bust to compress and flatten, thus creating the fashionable flat-chested garçonne silhouette. Origin: French—"bandage."

batiste (ba-tEst)
A sheer, light-weight woven fabric of linen or fine quality mercerized cotton. It was used for blouses, dresses, lingerie, and men's shirts.

baton (ba-ton)
The baton-link carrying chain was used for handbags and vanity cases. It contained alternate links which resembled slender metal bars or sticks. Origin: French—"stick."

beadlite
Introduced in the late 20s, beadlite was a variation of armor mesh containing small dome-shaped links resembling beads. Beadlite purses were often enameled.

belle époque, la (bel A-puk, lah)
French expression meaning "the beautiful era," circa 1895 to the First World War. This included the reign of Edward VII (1901-1910) which was a period of extravagant parties, dinners, and balls.

bias cut
A method of cutting garment pieces. Instead of placing the pattern pieces so that the warp threads run vertically and the weft threads run horizontally, pattern pieces are turned slightly so that the warp and weft threads are both on the diagonal. This gives the fabric a natural elasticity causing it to cling to the contours of the body. The bias cut required soft supple fabrics such as silk satin, silk velvet, crepe de chine, and chiffon. This was a favorite technique used by French couturiere Madeleine Vionnet.

bishop sleeve
A long set-in sleeve which is full from the elbow down, then gathered into a cuff at the wrist. Origin: a bishop's ecclesiastical garment.

boat neckline
A shallow, slightly curved neckline resembling a

boat. Also called a *bateau* (bah-tO) neckline, which means boat in French.

bouffant (bOO-fon)
French word for puffed out or full, as in the skirt of the robe de style.

boutonniere Fr. (bOO-tu-nE-Ar) / Eng. (bOO-tun-nEr)
A single fresh flower placed in the buttonhole of a man's lapel. Origin: French—"buttonhole."

brisé (brE-zA)
A type of fan with no pleated leaf. Instead a ribbon is laced through slits in the top of each overlapping blade holding them in the correct position. Origin: French—"broken to pieces."

brocade
A luxurious fabric with a raised pattern woven in, created on a special Jacquard loom. The pattern is produced by the incorporation of several different weaves which include the satin, rib, plain, and twill weaves. This fabric is not reversible as it has "floats" or loose threads running across the reverse side.

broché (bru-shA)
A heavy brocade fabric used for corsets and bandeaux during the 1920s.

brogue (brOg)
A sturdy low-heeled oxford with small perforations called broguings arranged in decorative patterns. Origin: Irish/Scotch country shoe.

broguings (brOg-ings)
Small decorative perforations in the leather found on various types of shoes including brogues, spectators, and saddle shoes. Also called punched leather. Origin: Scottish.

bugle beads
Small tubular glass beads produced in various lengths. They can be opaque, transparent, silver-lined, iridescent, or pearlized.

cabochon (ka-bo-shon)
A jewelry term for an unfaceted dome-shaped stone. Origin: French—"fancy brass nail."

Callot Soeurs (ka-lO ser)
The Callot sisters owned one of Paris' leading couture houses from 1916 to 1937. Their father was an antique dealer and supplied them with exquisite antique laces which they incorporated in their ultra feminine evening fashions. They were also the first to use gold and silver lamé. Origin: French—*soeurs*, "sisters."

carnival glass
Iridescent glass used for beads. It was made in America from 1910-1930.

cartouche (kar-tOOsh)
A French term for a small, smooth, geometric-shaped area (often raised slightly) on the surface of a metal object designed for an engraved monogram.

celluloid
An early form of plastic made of guncotton and camphor. This highly flammable substance was dyed to look like ivory, tortoise shell, coral, or amber.

challis (shal-E)
This light-weight plain-weave worsted has a soft brushed surface. It was a popular fabric for dresses and is usually printed in a mini floral or geometric pattern. Also spelled *challie, challys,* or *challi.* Origin: Anglo-Indian—"shalee."

chambray (shom-brA)
Smooth cotton fabric made by weaving white or unbleached threads across a colored warp.

chamois Fr. (sha-mwah) / Eng. (sha-mE)
Buff colored skin from the chamois antelope of the European mountains.

champlevé Fr. (shom-luh-vA) / Eng. (sham-plu-vA)
An enameling technique in which a design is carved or routed out of a metal object to form a shallow cavity. This cavity is then filled with enamel.

Chanel, Gabrielle "Coco"
Chanel was the most influential fashion designer of the 1920s. She adapted men's clothing into casual stylish fashions for women. She is noted for her classic suits, jersey dresses, costume jewelry, cardigan sweaters, beach pajamas, and her "little black dress."

Chantilly lace Fr. (shon-tE-yE) / Eng. (shan-til-E)
A delicate bobbin lace consisting of flowers and scrolls outlined with *cordonnet* on hexagonal mesh. Origin: the French town of Chantilly where this lace was first made.

Chelsea collar
A long pointed collar attached to a deep V-neckline.

chenille Fr. (shun-nE-yah) / Eng. (shun-nEl)
Soft fuzzy yarn with the feel of velvet. This two-ply yarn is twisted with short fluffy 1/8 inch threads caught between the plies and protruding from them to form a pile. A favorite fabric for bathrobes and bedspreads. Origin: French—"caterpillar."

Cheviot (shu-vE-yO)
Heavy wool twill fabric made from the fleece of Cheviot sheep. Origin: Cheviot hills between England and Scotland where these sheep were raised.

chignon (shEn-yon)
A bun or coil of hair at the nape of the neck. Origin: French.

chiné (shEn-A)
A French term for the Chinese textile printing technique in which the warp or vertical threads are printed before the fabric is woven. This creates a design with a soft blurred effect.

chiton (kI-ten)
A simple ancient Greek garment made from a large rectangle of linen fabric. The fabric was folded in half (with the fold running vertically on one side) creating a front and a back. These two sides were fastened together over each shoulder with 4-5 *fibula* (decorative pins). When the chiton was girdled at the waist, a long sleeved effect was produced. The Greek chiton was an inspiration for the "delphos" dresses designed by Mariano Fortuny.

chou (shOO) pl. choux (shOO)
A large fabric rosette used as a trimming. Origin: French—"cabbage, rosette."

civet cat (sE-vA)
Cat-like flesh eating mammal with gray and black spotted fur. Origin: French—*civette.*

cloche Fr. (klush) / Eng. (klOsh)
Bell-shaped hat with deep snug fitting crown and narrow brim. It covered the forehead in front and the hair to the nape of the neck in back. Origin: French—"bell."

cloisonné Fr. (klwa-zO-nA) / Eng. (cloy-zO-nA)
An ancient enameling technique used to decorate the surface of a metal object. Fine wire is bent to form a design which is fastened to the surface of the object. This forms shallow compartments which are each filled with a different colored enamel. Origin: French—*cloison* "partition."

coutil (kOO-tE)
Sturdy cotton twill fabric, used for foundation garments. Also spelled *coutille.* Origin: French—"ticking."

couture (kOO-tOOr)
French term for original custom-made styles, handmade from the finest fabrics by noted designers. Origin: French—"sewing, needlework."

couture (kOO-tOOr) house
The headquarters of a French fashion designer which could include show rooms, fitting rooms, and an *atelier* (ah-tel-E-A) or workroom.

couturier (kOO-tOOr-E-A)
French term for male fashion designer.

couturiere (kOO-tOOr-E-Ar)
French term for female fashion designer.

crepe Fr. (krep) / Eng. (krape)
A fabric with a pebbly surface made from highly twisted threads. Origin: French.

crepe de chine Fr. (krep-duh-shEn) / Eng. (krape duh shEn)
Fine light-weight low-luster crepe fabric made of raw silk. Highly twisted weft threads are used and more warp than weft threads. Used for lingerie, dresses, and blouses. Origin: French "crepe of China."

Cubism
An art movement of the early 20th century, in which the subject was reduced to the simplest geometric forms. Shapes were used in abstract arrangements rather than realistic representations of nature. Cubism was an important influence on the Art Deco movement. Origin: French—*cubisme.*

cummerbund
A wide cloth sash worn as a waistband for a dress or with a men's tuxedo. Origin: Hindi/Persian—*Kamarband* "loin band."

Delaunay (de-lO-nA), Sonia
Russian-born painter/designer who created fashions from printed fabrics which she created herself. Her bold Cubistic designs featured abstract geometric shapes rendered in vivid hues, usually on a white background.

de rigueur (duh rE-ger)
French term meaning necessary, compulsory, a must.

diamanté (dE-ah-mon-tA)
Diamond-like sparkling stones such as rhinestones. Origin: French—"made of diamonds."

Doucet, Jacques (dOO-sA, zhok)
Well known designer who opened his Paris couture house c.1875. He designed for actresses, socialites, and royalty. He favored the use of lace, iridescent silks, and fur trim.

engine turnings
Decorative machine engraving on metal objects such as jewelry, compacts, vanities, cigarette cases and lighters. Typical patterns were rows of dots, circles, squares, waves, and stripes. Also popular were sunrays, basket weaves, concentric circles, and kaleidoscopes.

fagoting
Fancy crisscross embroidery stitches (like tiny connecting bridges) which stretch across a 1/4 inch gap between the parallel edges of two pieces of fabric. Fagoting provides a decorative more supple alternative to the common seam.

faience (fah-E-ons)
Colorful glazed pottery beads used by Egyptians in the creation of dramatic necklaces, earrings, and bracelets. Origin: French—"earthenware."

faille Fr. (fl-yah) / Eng. (file)
Ribbed fabric of silk, rayon, cotton, or wool. It was used for women's dresses, suits, and coats; as well as the lapels and trouser stripes of men's tails and tuxedos. Origin: French.

Fauvism (fOv-ism)
A expressionist art style characterized by bold distortions and bright colors. Henri Matisse and André Derain were noted French fauvist painters. Origin: French—*Les Fauves* "the wild beasts."

faux (fO)
French term meaning false, fake, or synthetic.

filigree
Jewelry made of fine wire twisted into delicate lacy openwork resembling lace. By the 1920s, filigree work was die cast from white gold, sterling, brass, nickel, and base metal. Origin: French—*filigrane.*

fleur-de-lis (fler-duh-lE)
This royal emblem of France, introduced in the 12th century, was patterned after the iris. Origin: French—"flower of lily."

flounce
Horizontal strip of fabric, gathered at the top and stitched to a skirt (usually at the hem). Can be single or multiple rows.

fontanges (fon-tonzh)
A form of headdress popularized by the Duchesses of Fontanges, mistress of Louis XIV (1680). It consisted of a pleated piece of starched lace resembling a partially opened fan with rounded corners. It was attached to the top of a lace cap so that it stood up vertically.

Fortuny, Mariano
Fortuny is noted for his classical "Delphos" dresses made of diaphanous pleated silk in soft muted shades. The edges were weighted with handmade Venetian glass beads. To accompany these dresses, he designed silk velvet evening wraps, which he printed with gold and silver paint in patterns reminiscent of medieval and Renaissance tapestries.

full fashion marks
Small desirable dots or marks in the knit along the seams of hosiery. They were caused by increasing or decreasing stitches.

gaiters
Felt, cloth, or leather coverings extending from mid-calf to the bottom of the shoe. They were buttoned down the outside of the leg and were fastened under the instep with buckled straps. Also called *spats* or *leggings*. They began to disappear in the late teens.

galosh
Waterproof mid-calf boot worn over the shoe, featuring hinged metal fasteners (which flappers preferred to leave open). Also called an Arctic boot or overshoe. Also spelled *galoshe* or *golosh*. Origin: French—*galoche* "clog."

garçonne (gar-sun)
French word for boy (garçon), but with a feminine ending. Used to describe the desirable flat-chested boyish figure of 1920s flappers.

gauntlet
A glove with wide flared cuff above the wrist, reminiscent of the gloves worn by 17th century Musketeers. Origin: French.

gazelle
Small swift antelope which, because of its speed, became a popular Art Deco motif.

georgette or georgette crepe
Thin loosely-woven plain-weave fabric made of highly twisted yarn. It is heavier than chiffon with a pebbly texture. It was a popular fabric for dresses and gowns during the 1920s. Origin: Named after Georgette de la Plante, a Parisian milliner.

gillie oxford
This Scottish dancing shoe, originally worn with a kilt, was introduced in the United States by the Prince of Wales. It had no tongue and was laced through leather loops rather than eyelets. Also called the *Prince of Wales shoe*.

godet (gO-dA)
Triangular-shaped pieces of fabric inserted into the hem of a dress to add a slight flare. Diamond-shaped godets were also used creating a pointed hem.

grosgrain (grO-grAn)
Ribbon with a rib created by placing filling threads together in groups.

guilloché (gE-yO-shA) enameling
Decorative treatment used on metal objects. Engine turnings (machine engravings) were covered with a layer of translucent enamel which allowed the engraved grooves to show through.

gunmetal
A form of bronze, gunmetal is an alloy of 90% copper and 10% tin. It melts readily and is easily molded. It is also resistant to rust. It is bluish/gray in color and can be polished to a fine, smooth finish. It became popular for jewelry and handbag frames in the 1890s.

hand-tooled leather
Leather that has been stamped with a metal die (tool) producing an impressed design. Each individual portion of the main design was stamped by hand.

haute couture (O-tuh kOO-tOOr)
High fashion. Origin: French—feminine form of *haut*—"high."

Heim, Jacques (hIm, zhok)
French designer who joined the family fur business in 1923. He built the house into a world-famous couture establishment by designing chic, high fashion fur coats for his distinctive clientele.

hemstitching
An openwork embroidery treatment in which two or three parallel threads are snipped and removed from the fabric. The cross threads are then pulled together in groups of 3s or 4s using embroidery stitches. (When hemstitching is cut down the center, it creates two picot edges.)

huarache (wah-rah-cha)
A shoe made of closely woven leather thongs. Origin: Mexican—"woven low-heeled slingback sandal."

infanta
Any daughter of a King of Spain or Portugal, often depicted in 17th century portraits wearing formal gowns with ultra-wide skirts.

jabot (zha-bO)
Decorative vertical ruffle attached to the neck of a lady's blouse or dress. Origin: French—"frill."

japan
A varnish which creates a hard glossy finish. Origin: Japan.

jersey
Soft, elastic, knitted cloth featuring the V-shaped knit stitch. Chanel was the first to use lowly wool jersey as a dress fabric, which caused Paul Poiret to call her designs "the deluxe poor look." Origin: the British Isle of Jersey in the English Channel where it was first produced.

jodhpurs (jod-perz)
Riding breeches popular after World War I. They billowed out in a semicircle over the hips, then fit snugly from the knees down. Origin: Jodhpur is a city in India.

kiltie oxford
Sport shoe with tasseled laces which tie over a fringed tongue. Origin: an adaptation of a Scottish shoe.

lamé (la-mA)
Woven fabric of gold or silver metallic thread. Origin: French— "silver or gold leaves."

lampwork beads (lamp beads)
Each fancy lampwork bead was made individually by hand. A colored glass "cane" or rod was heated over a lamp flame until the end became malleable. The softened end was wound around a copper wire (which produced the center hole), then rolled in a mold to perfect the shape. "Goldstone" or aventurine glass, containing small particles of mica or copper, created a glittery effect. Small pink rosebuds were added to beads by coiling a piece of molten cane onto the surface of the bead. Spirals were also added by trailing molten glass over the bead while it was turned. Lampwork beads were produced in Gablonz, Czechoslovakia, and on the island of Murano, near Venice, Italy.

Lanvin, Jeanne (lon-van, zhan)
Lanvin is noted for her bouffant "robe de style" dresses resembling the 18th century "robe a la française." She is also remembered for her mother and daughter dresses.

lapis lazuli Fr. (la-pEs la-zOO-lE) / Eng. (la-pis la-zOO-lE)
An opaque gemstone of deep-blue color, often with white mottlings.

layette (lA-yet)
Garments and accessories assembled for the newborn including diapers, sacques, undershirts, towels, and washcloths.

lingerie Fr. (lan-zha-rE) / Eng. (lon-gu-rA)
Ladies' intimate apparel including undergarments and sleepwear. Origin: French—*linge*, "linen."

lisle (lEl)
Two-ply hardspun cotton yarn which was used for stockings and socks in the early part of the 20th century. Eventually replaced by silk and rayon. Origin: French town of Lille.

Louiseboulanger (lOO-Ez-bOO-lon-zhA)
Combined her names Louise and Boulanger. She opened her couture house in 1923. She is known for her ultra-chic bias-cut styles and sophisticated bi-level gowns.

macramé (ma-kra-mA)
Decorative knotting technique used on fringe shawls.

madras
Handwoven Indian cotton usually made in plaids, stripes, or checks. The vegetable-dyed yarns "bled" when washed giving the fabric a softer, more muted look. Origin: Madras, India, where it was originally made.

mah-jongg
A game of Chinese origin, played with small tiles. This game was all the rage in the 1920s.

mantilla (man-tE-yah)
Spanish shawl or veil usually made of black or white lace. It was draped over a high back comb and allowed to fall over the shoulders. Origin: Spanish—*manta*, "shawl."

marabou
Soft fluffy under plumage from the wings and tail of the African marabou stork. It was used to trim negligees and boudoir slippers during the 1920s.

marcasite (mar-ka-zIt)
Crystallized white iron pyrite, used as an inexpensive substitute for diamonds. It is opaque, and therefore obtains its sparkle from the light reflected from its facets.

Marcel
In 1872, a French hair dresser named Marcel Grateau invented a technique for waving the hair by the use of a curling iron. The "marcel wave," as it was later called, reached the height of popularity during the 20s and 30s.

mercerization
A process developed by John Mercer, a calico dyer from Lancashire, England, in 1844. It involves the treatment of cotton threads or fabric with caustic soda, which gives it a permanent silky luster. It also increases its softness, strength, and receptivity to dyes.

mirror-image clasp
A two part clasp with one side the reverse reflection of the other.

moiré Fr. (mwa-rA) / Eng. (mor-A)
Fabric with a watery-effect produced by the use of heated pressure rollers.

Molyneux, Edward (mOl-E-nOz, ed-war)
This English-Irish designer is noted for his tailored wool and printed silk suits, and matching ensembles.

Mondrian, Piet (mon-drE-an, pEt)
Cubist painter who created abstract paintings which featured blocks of primary color separated by black grid lines.

monobosom
The large low-slung matronly bosom which had the appearance of one hump (not two). This look was very desirable at the turn of the century and constituted the top half of the "S-bend" figure.

nainsook (nAn-sook)
Soft light-weight plain-weave cotton fabric. Origin: Hindi.

necessaire **(nes-ses-air)**
A small cylindrical-shaped vanity case with compartments for some of the following items: makeup, cigarettes, handkerchief, comb, money, slate, celluloid, pencil, or bobby pins. They were suspended from a silk wrist cord or carrying chain and usually ended with a tassel which frequently concealed a tube of lipstick. Origin: French—"necessary."

negligee Fr. (neg-lE-zhA) / Eng. (neg-luh-zhA)
Flowing robe of sheer fabric, trimmed with ruffles, feathers, or lace. Usually worn over a matching nightgown. Also called a *dressing gown.*

Norfolk suit
This sporty jacket featured four box pleats (two in front and two in back) with slots so that the matching belt could be slipped under each pleat. It was worn with long pants or knickers.

nutria
South American water dwelling rodent with short soft brown fur, and webbed feet. Origin: Spanish.

paillette **(pA-yet)**
Metal spangle, slightly larger than a sequin, used to decorate evening dresses and bandeaux.

pannier **(pan-yA)**
Eighteenth century wire, whale bone, or wicker undergarment worn over the hips to support the wide skirt of the robe á la française. Origin: French—"baskets."

parure **(par-OOr)**
A matching set of jewelry consisting of a necklace, earrings, bracelet, brooch, ring, and occasionally a tiara. Less than a complete set is known as a demi-parure. Origin: French—"finery, ornament."

patina
The natural discoloration of an object caused by aging. Origin: French—*patine.*

Patou, Jean (pa-tOO, zhon)
French designer who is known for his wearable sports clothing, i.e. tennis outfits for Suzanne Lenglen and sweaters with Cubist designs. He was responsible for lowering the hemline in 1929 to mid-calf for day and the ankle for evening. He also raised the waist to its normal position that same year.

percale
Light-weight plain-weave fabric made of fine combed cotton.

Peter Pan collar
Small round collar curving up to the neck at center front.

petit point Fr. (pe-tE pwan) / Eng. (pe-tE point)
Embroidery which consists of rows of diagonal stitches on a grid-work canvas is called *needlepoint.* Petit point contains smaller stitches. Origin: French.

picot (pE-kO)
1. Rows of tiny loops along the selvage of picot ribbon or the edge of certain laces. 2. A machine-made edging on a garment containing a row of tiny tufts resembling picots. This edging is usually used on sheer fabric in lieu of the stiffer folded hem.

Pierrot (pE-ehr-O) collar
Large ruffled collar attached to a jewel neckline. Origin: patterned after the costume of Pierrot, the French pantomime comedian.

pince-nez **(panc-nA)**
Eyeglasses without temples, held in place by a spring-tension nose piece. Origin: French "pinch nose."

piqué **(pE-kA)**
Crisp fabric made with cords causing a raised rib or honeycomb effect. Origin: French.

placket
A slit at the neck, waistband, or wrist designed for ease in dressing and undressing.

plissé **(plE-sA)**
A cotton fabric with a puckered finish.

pochette **(posh-et)**
A flat rectangular bag which reached its peak of popularity in the late 20s and 30s. It resembled an envelope with a flap or contained a metal frame with a top clasp. *Pochettes* contained either a short horizontal top strap, or a vertical back strap. These bags were either carried by the top strap, tucked under the arm or clutched in the hand.

Poiret (pwa-ray), Paul
French couturier who dominated the fashion scene from 1909 to 1924. He was influenced by the vivid colors and Oriental styles of the Ballet Russe. He designed sumptuous eastern-style tunics with kimono or dolman sleeves, exotic turbans decked with aigrettes, and "lampshade" dresses. He banished the corset, but shackled the ankles with his narrow "hobble" skirts.

polychromatic
Multi-colored.

pongee
A plain-weave fabric made from wild silk usually in its natural ecru color. The weft threads are irregular in thickness, creating slubs. Origin: Chinese—*pen-chi* "home loom."

plastron
A piece of fabric inserted into the V, U, or square-shaped neckline of a blouse or dress. The plastron was often decorated or made of a contrasting color or texture.

protégé Mas. (prO-tA-zhA)
protégée Fem. (prO-tA-zhA)
A person receiving guidance from an influential person on furthering his/her career. Origin: French.

punchwork
Openwork embroidery in which threads are pulled aside and fastened with decorative stitches. Also called *pullwork.*

rayon
A synthetic fiber made from cellulose which was pressed through small holes to form filaments. Called artificial silk until 1924, when it was renamed rayon. It draped well and accepted dye readily, however, it wrinkled easily and often shrunk with washing.

Reboux (re-bOO), Caroline
The leading French milliner who introduced the *cloche* hat (c. 1923), the gigolo hat (c. 1925), and elegant lamé turbans.

reticule
Pouch style handbag with a drawstring top, formerly made of net. Origin: French—"netlike."

robe à la française (rub ah lah fron-sez)
An elegant 18th century gown featuring a triangular stomacher, an oval skirt with wide extended sides, and a loose back with box pleats which hang from the shoulders. Origin: French style gown.

rocaille (rO-kl)
Also called Indian beads, these tiny glass beads can be transparent, translucent, opaque, pearlized, iridescent, or foil lined. They were used to decorate gowns, bandeaux, bags, shoes, blouses, and jewelry.

Rococo
The delicate 18th century decorative style which featured flowers, foliage, shell work, and scrolls.

ruching (rOO-shing)
Trim which resembles a ruffle. It consists of a strip of fabric, lace, ribbon, or net which is pleated width-wise and stitched down the center to a garment.

sacque (sack)
A loose fitting garment hanging from the shoulders.

sautoir (sO-twa)
A long necklace terminating with a tassel. Origin: French.

sans-serif (son-su-rEf)
French term which refers to printed type or letters which have no serifs or fine lines projecting from the main stroke of the letter. Origin: French.

sateen
A smooth glossy cotton fabric made to look like satin.

S-bend silhouette
The ideal feminine figure of the turn of the century which (when viewed from the side) resembled the letter "S." It consisted of a large low-slung mono-bosom, a wasp waist, and a large rear.

scarab
1. The black winged dung beetle, a sacred Egyptian symbol of life. 2. An image cut from stone to resemble a beetle, frequently used in 1920s jewelry.

scarf pin
Decorative pin containing an ornamental top on the end of a pointed shaft. The top was usually set with faceted stones or a cabochon. It was inserted vertically into a necktie with a clutch or guard placed on the opposite end for safety. It was also called a *tie pin* or *stick pin*.

Schiaparelli (Skap-a-rel-E), Elsa
Italian born designer who began her career, in 1928, with her *trompe l'oeil* sweaters. She loved to shock and her 1930s fashions often featured surrealistic ideas contributed by such artists as Dali and Cocteau.

scoop neckline
Broad, round, open neckline.

selvage
The side edges of a piece of fabric where the weft threads wrap around the warp threads to prevent unraveling. Origin: formerly "self edge."

serge
A smooth durable fabric made with worsted yarns in the twill weave. Used for suits, skirts, and trousers.

shantung
A silk fabric with an uneven surface made of thread with elongated slubs. Origin: Shantung, China, where it was first produced.

shawl collar
A long gently-curved one-piece collar without notches. It is attached to a V-neckline and tapers to a point at the bottom.

shirring
Parallel rows of gathering stitches.

surplice Fr. (sOOr-plEs) / Eng. (sur-plis)
A crisscrossed bodice consisting of two overlapping sides with diagonal upper edges which create a V-neckline. Origin: French.

taffeta
A crisp stiff plain-weave fabric made of silk or rayon with an iridescent luster. Its stiffness made it an ideal fabric for the full-skirted robe de style. Origin: Persian—*taftan* "to weave."

tailleur (tI-yer)
1. A tailor. 2. Women's two-piece suit. Origin: French.

tiers
Layers of straight or bias cut ruffles which overlap each other. Used mainly on skirts.

toque (tOk)
Small round brimless hat, perched on the top of the head. Popular from the 1890s through the very early twenties. Origin: French—"jockey's cap."

tricorne hat
A hat introduced for men in the late 17th century. It featured a wide brim, cocked on three sides forming three points. Also spelled *tricorn*. Origin: French—*corne*, "horn."

trompe l'oeil (tromp loy)
Any design element or detail which is deceiving to the eye, i.e. the trompe l'oeil sweaters designed by Elsa Schiaparelli. Origin: French—"trick of the eye."

tulle (tool)
Fine sheer net with hexagonal holes. It was left unstarched for bridal veils and starched for bouffant skirts. Origin: the city of Tulle, France, where it was made.

tuxedo collar
Similar to the shawl collar, but retaining the same width down the full length of the garment.

Valenciennes lace (va-lon-sE-yen)
A bobbin lace characterized by small flower and bow motifs on a background of diamond-shaped mesh. Origin: the French town of Valenciennes where it was first made. *Val lace*—the abbreviation for Valenciennes lace. This term usually refers to machine-made lace.

vicuña (vI-kOOn-yah)
The soft, strong fiber of the South American vicuña, a member of the llama family. Dark brown or fawn in color, it was used for coats, jackets, and suits.

Vionnet (vE-O-nA), Madeleine
One of the most influential French designers, Vionnet set the trend for bias cut dresses and other garments in the late 20s and 30s. The suppleness of the fabrics and the elasticity of bias cut allowed her garments to be pulled over the head without fastenings.

voile Fr. (vwal) / Eng. (voil)
Fine sheer open-weave fabric of tightly-twisted threads. It was made of cotton and used for blouses and dresses. Origin: French *veil*, "veil."

Vuitton, Louis (vwE-ton, lOO-E)
Founder of the world's most prestigious luggage firm. This concern made baggage for the Empress Eugenie in the mid 19th century. The company logo consists of yellow LVs and *fleurons* (flowers) on a brown background.

BIBLIOGRAPHY

Allen, Frederick Lewis. *Only Yesterday*. New York: Harper and Row, 1964.

Baclawski, Karen. *The Guide to Historic Costume*. New York: Drama Book Publishers, 1995.

Baker, Lillian. *Art Nouveau and Art Deco Jewelry*. Paducah: Collector Books, 1981.

_____. *One Hundred Years of Collectible Jewelry*. Paducah: Collector Books, 1978.

_____. *Twentieth Century Fashionable Plastic Jewelry*. Paducah: Collector Books, 1992.

Ball, Joanne and Dorothy Torem. *The Art of Fashion Accessories*. Atglen: Schiffer Publishing Ltd., 1993.

Batterberry, Michael and Ariane. *Fashion the Mirror of History*. New York: Greenwich House, 1977.

Battersby, Martin. *Art Deco Fashion: French Designers 1908-1925*. London: Academy Editions, 1974.

Battle, Dee and Alayne Lesser. *The Best of Bakelite and Other Plastic Jewelry*. Atglen: Schiffer Publishing, Ltd., 1996.

Becker, Vivienne. *Fabulous Costume Jewelry: History of Fantasy and Fashion in Jewels*. Atglen: Schiffer Publishing Ltd., 1993.

Black, J. Anderson and Madge Garland (updated and revised by France Kennett). *A History of Fashion*. London: Orbis, 1980.

Blum, Stella. *Everyday Fashions of the Twenties: As Pictured in Sears and Other Catalogs*. New York: Dover Publications, Inc., 1981.

Bronson, Louis D. *Early American Specs*. Glendale: The Occidental Publishing Company, 1974.

Byrde, Penelope. *A Visual History of Costume: The Twentieth Century*. London: B.T. Batsford Ltd., 1987.

Calasibetta, Charlotte Mankey. *Fairchild's Dictionary of Fashion*. New York: Fairchild Publications, 1988.

Carter, Alison. *Underwear: The Fashion History*. New York: Drama Book Publishers, 1992.

Carter, Ernestine. *The Changing World of Fashion*. New York: G.P. Putnam's Sons, 1977.

Charles-Roux, Edmonde. *Chanel and Her World*. London: The Vendome Press, 1981.

Coles, Janet and Robert Budwig. *The Book of Beads*. New York: Simon and Schuster, 1990.

Corson, Richard. *Fashions in Eyeglasses*. Chester Springs: Dufour Editions, Ins., 1967.

Cumming, Valerie. *The Costume Accessories Series: Gloves*. London: B.T. Batsford Ltd., 1982.

Cunnington, C. Willett and Phillis. *The History of Underclothes*. London: Faber and Faber, 1981.

Davidson, D.C. *Spectacles, Lorgnettes and Monocles*. Buckinghamshire: Shire Publications, 1989.

De Courtais, Georgine. *Women's Headdresses and Hairstyles*. London: B.T. Batsford Ltd., 1973.

Deslandres, Yvonne. *Poiret*. New York: Rizzoli, 1987.

de Osma, Guillermo. *Mariano Fortuny: His Life and Work*. New York: Rizzoli, 1985.

Donner, Kate. *A Century of Handbags*. Atglen: Schiffer Publishing Ltd., 1993.

Eckstein, E. and J. and G. Firkins. *Gentlemen's Dress Accessories*. Buckinghamshire: Shire Publications Ltd., 1987.

Ettinger, Roseann. *Compacts and Smoking Accessories*. Atglen: Schiffer Publishing Ltd., 1991.

_____. *Handbags*. Atglen: Schiffer Publishing Ltd., 1991.

_____. *Popular Jewelry: 1840-1940*. Atglen: Schiffer Publishing Ltd., 1990.

Ewing, Elizabeth. *Dress and Undress*. London: Bibliophine, 1978.

Farrell, Jeremy. *The Costume Accessories Series: Socks and Stockings*. London: B.T. Batsford Limited, 1992.

_____. *The Costume Accessories Series: Umbrellas and Parasols*. London: B.T. Batsford Limited, 1985.

Foster, Vanda. *The Costume Accessories Series: Bags and Purses*. London: B.T. Batsford Limited, 1982.

Gerson, Roselyn. *Vintage Vanity Bags & Purses*. Paducah: Collector Books, 1994.

Ginsburg, Madeleine. *Paris Fashions: The Art Deco Style of the 1920s*. London: Bracken Books, 1989.

Glennon, Lorraine (ed.) *Our Times: The Illustrated History of the 20th Century*. Atlanta: Turner Publishing, Inc., 1995.

Glynn, Prudence. *In Fashion: Dress in the Twentieth Century*. New York: Oxford University Press, 1978.

Gold, Annalee. *Seventy Five Years of Fashion*. New York: Fairchild Publications, 1975.

Hall, Lee. *Common Threads: A Parade of American Clothing*. Boston: Bulfinch Press, 1992.

Herald, Jacqueline. *Fashions of a Decade: the 1920s*. New York: Facts on File, 1991.

Houck, Catherine. *The Fashion Encyclopedia*. New York: St. Martin's Press, 1982.

Jargstorf, Sibylle. *Baubles, Buttons and Beads: The Heritage of Bohemia*. Atglen: Schiffer Publishing Ltd., 1993.

Kelly, Lyngerda and Nancy Schiffer. *Plastic Jewelry*. Atglen: Schiffer Publishing Ltd., 1987.

Kennett, Frances. *The Collector's Book of Fashion*. New York: Crown Publishers, Inc., 1983.

Lansdell, Avril. *History in Camera: Seaside Fashions 1860-1939*. Buckinghamshire: Shire Publications Ltd., 1990.

Lansdell, Avril. *History in Camera: Wedding Fashions 1860-1980*. Buckinghamshire: Shire Publications Ltd., 1983.

Laver, James. *Costume & Fashion: A Concise History*. New York: Oxford University Press, 1982.

_____. *Modesty in Dress*. Boston: Houghton Mifflin Company, 1969.

Lynnlee, J.L. *All That Glitters*. Atglen: Schiffer Publishing Ltd., 1986.

Mackrell, Alice. *CoCo Chanel*. New York: Holmes & Meier, 1992.

_____. *The Costume Accessories Series: Shawls, Stoles and Scarves*. London: B.T. Batsford Ltd., 1986.

_____. *Paul Poiret*. London: B.T. Batsford Ltd., 1990.

McDowell, Colin. *Shoes: Fashion and Fantasy*. New York: Rizzoli, 1989.

Menten, Theodore. *The Art Deco Style*. New York: Dover Publications, Inc. 1922.

Mueller, Laura M. *Collector's Encyclopedia of Compacts, Carryalls, & Face Powder Boxes*. Paducah: Collector Books, 1994.

Mulvagh, Jane. *Costume Jewelry in Vogue*. New York: Thames and Hudson, 1988.

Newman, Harold. *An Illustrated Dictionary of Jewelry*. London: Thames and Hudson, 1981.

O'Hara, Georgina. *The Encyclopaedia of Fashion*. New York: Harry N. Abrams, Inc., Publishers, 1986.

Robins, Bill. *An A-Z of Gems and Jewelry*. New York: Arco Publishing, Inc., 1982.

Robinson, Julian. *The Golden Age of Style: Art Deco Fashion Illustration*. New York: Gallery Books, 1976.

Ross, Josephine. *Society in Vogue: The International Set Between the Wars*. New York: Vendome Press, 1992.

Schiffer, Nancy. *Handbook of Fine Jewelry*. Atglen: Schiffer Publishing Ltd., 1991.

Schoeffler, O.E. and William Dale. *Esquire's Encyclopedia of 20th Century Men's Fashion*. New York: McGraw Hill, 1973.

Schwartz, Lynell K. *Vintage Purses At Their Best*. Atglen: Schiffer Publishing Ltd., 1995.

Shields, Jody. *Hats: A Stylish History and Collector's Guide.* New York: Clarkson Potter Publishers, 1991.

Stegemeyer, Anne. *Who's Who In Fashion.* New York: Fairchild Publications, 1980.

Swann, June. *The Costume Accessories Series: Shoes.* London: B.T. Batsford Ltd., 1982.

Time-Life Editors. *This Fabulous Century: 1920-1930.* Alexandria: Time-Life Books, Inc., 1969.

Tortora, Phyllis and Keith Eubank. *Survey of Historic Costume.* New York: Fairchild Publications, 1994.

Tranquillo, Mary D. *Styles of Fashion: A Pictorial Handbook.* New York: Van Nostrand Reinhold Company, 1984.

Trasko, Mary. *Heavenly Soles: Extraordinary Twentieth-Century Shoes.* New York: Abbeville Press, 1989.

White, Palmer. *Elsa Schiaparelli: Empress of Paris Fashion.* New York: Rizzoli, 1986.

Wilcox, R. Turner. *The Dictionary of Costume.* New York: Charles Scribner's Sons, 1969.

_____. *The Mode in Costume.* New York: Charles Schribner's Sons, 1958.

_____. *The Mode in Footwear.* New York: Charles Scribner Sons, 1948.

Yarwood, Doreen. *Costume of the Western World.* St. New York: Martin's Press, 1980.

_____. *The Encyclopedia of Costume.* New York: Bonanza Books, 1978.

Zimmerman, Catherine. *The Bride's Book: A Pictorial History of American Bridal Gowns.* New York: Arbor House, 1985, pp. 198-205.

CATALOGS

Charles William Store, Inc., New York, Fall and Winter, 1927/1928.

Franklin Simon & Co., Fifth Avenue Fashions, Spring and Summer, 1926.

Hamilton Garment Co., New York, 1930.

Humania Hair and Specialty Mfg. Co., New York, 1926.

Jason Weiler-Baird North Co., Boston, Mass., 1929

John Wanamaker Store and Home, Philadelphia, Summer - 1929; Fall and Winter - 1921/1922.

Lane Bryant, New York, 1929.

Montgomery Ward & Co., Fall and Winter - 1920/1921

M.W. Savage Co., Chicago, Fall and Winter - 1927/1928.

National Bellas Hess Co., New York - 1928.

National Cloak & Suit Co., New York, Spring and Summer - 1927.

Sears, Roebuck and Co., Chicago, Spring and Summer - 1923; Fall and Winter - 1923; Spring and Summer - 1928/1929; Fall and Winter - 1928/1929.

Stewart & Co., New York, Fall and Winter - 1925/1926.

The Washington Jewelry Company, Boston, 1925.

PERIODICALS

Butterick Quarterly (Autumn 1922, Winter 1922-1923, Summer 1926).

Elite Magazine (4/1923).

Fashion Service Magazine (1928).

Harper's Magazine (4/1924).

McCall's (7/1926, 2/1927, 1/1928, 4/1928, 9/1928, 4/1929).

McCall Quarterly (Summer/1927).

Needle Art (1920).

Needlecraft Magazine (6/1925).

Pictorial Review (10/1925).

Reinach's Review of Fashion, Paris (6 issues - 1928).

Ribbon Art Book, (1923).

Town & Country (8/1922, 9/1922, 6/1925, 4/1926, 9/1926).

Weldon's Ladies Journal (8/29.)

Woman's Home Companion (6/1928).

Woman's Magazine (2/1920).

Vogue (1/1/25, 3/1/25, 5/1/25, 6/1/25, 10/1/25, 4/1/26, 5/1/26, 6/1/26, 7/15/26, 9/1/26, 9/15/26, 1/1/27, 2/15/27, 3/1/27, 4/1/27, 4/15/27, 8/15/27, 9/1/27, 3/1/28.)

Vogue Fashion Bi-Monthly (Feb/Mar 1927.)

PERIODICAL AND NEWSPAPER ARTICLES

Blue, Wendy. "Publicity in Hand: A Brief History of Folding Advertising Fans." *Lady's Gallery* (Feb/Mar 1995) 14-18.

Giunca, Mary. "Fortuny of Venice." *Lady's Gallery* (Oct/Nov 1995). 8-13.

Haertig, Evelyn. "The Purse in History." *Lady's Gallery* (Nov-Dec 1995) 28-31.

LaMothe, Terri L. "Art Deco and the Mesh Bag: 1919-1930." *Lady's Gallery* (June/July 1995) 16-21.

Mc Cormick, "Hats Complete the Total Fashion Look." *Antique Week* 22 (14 Aug 1989), 1 and 48.

McAlister, Wilda. "Curling Irons - For Men, Too." *Spinning Wheel* (Jan/Feb 1976) 29-32.

Watson, Bruce. "In the Heyday of Men's Hats, Fashion Began at the Top." *Smithsonian* (March 1994). 73-81.

PRICE GUIDE

Prices vary greatly according to the craftmanship, overall design, size, color, condition, rarity, and the intrinsic value of the materials. Current fashion trends and the location of the market may also be determining factors. The price ranges offered here reflect these variations and are merely a guide.

The column on the left indicates the page number. The letters correspond to the location of the item on the page:

TL= top left   TC= top center   TR=top right
CL=center right   C=center   CR=center right
BL=bottom left   BC=bottom   BR=bottom right

The column on the right suggests the price range in United States dollars.

For practical reasons, we will assume that all of the items in this price guide are in good condition.

Page	Loc	Price	Page	Loc	Price	Page	Loc	Price
17	TL	2-5	33	TL	35-50	53	BR	150-200
		15-25		BL	150-200	54	CL	75-100
		15-20	34	TR	75-95		C	150-200
18	CL	15-25		BC	50-75			200-300
	BL	20-25		BR	50-75	57	TL	75-100
20	TL	20-40	35	TL	40-68	59	TL	100-150
	CL	25-35		BR	40-60	60	BR	150-175
	TC	15-30	37	TR	50-75	61	TR	175-250
	BC	35-50		CL	40-50	62	C	90-100
21	TL	15-30	38	TL	50-70		BL	125-150
	CL	10-20		TR	75-90	64	TR	150-175
	C	20-30		BL	150-175		BL	60-80
	TR	25-35		BR	75-100	65	TL	125-150
22	TL	25-35	44	TC	250-325		TR	15-25
	TR	10-20		TR	7,000-10,000	66	BR	100-150
	BL	10-15	45	TR	500-600	67	CL	75-125
	BR	10-50		BL	400-600	68	BR	40-50
23	TL	40-50	46	TL	350-450	69	BL	15-25
	TR	2-5		TR	250-350			50-75
24	CL	70-90		BL	300-400		BR	25-40
		125-175		BR	75-100	70	BL	40-50
		70-90	47	BL	50-75	71	BR	15-35
	BC	50-70	48	CL	125-150	72	CL	20-40
	BR	40-60		TL	125-175			50-75
25		35-50		TR	100-150		CR	50-60
26	TR	75-100		BL	175-200			20-25
	C	110-140		BR	75-100	77	CL	100-150
	CR	300-800	50	BL	300-400		BC	125-175
27	TL	35-50		BC	400-450		BR	275-325
	CL	20-30	51	TL	500-600	79	TL	275-350
	CR	50-75		TR	175-200	81	C	250-300
28	BL	2-5	52	TL	250-300		CR	50-75
31	TR	75-125		TR	250-300	82	CL	275-300
	BL	50-70		BL	275-300		CR	275-300

85	TR	15-25	101	TL	40-50	116	TL	400-500
	BL	25-50	102	TR	275-375		CL	500-700
	BR	15-25		BL	350-450		CR	450-600
86	TL	10-20	103	TL	70-120	117	TL	400-500
		15-25		TR	80-130		BL	400-500
	TR	5-15/set		BL	80-130	118	BL	500-600
	BL	5-20/set		BR	70-120	119	TL	100-150
		5-20/set	104	TR	100-135		TR	125-200
89	TR	100-125			150-175		CL	150-200
	BL	75-100		CL	110-140		BR	100-190
	BR	75-100		BR	150-175	120	TL	100-175
90	TL	60-90	105	TL	100-150		TR	100-150
	CL	50-80		TR	100-125		CL	80-120
	CR	50-75		BL	100-125		BR	150-250
		85-100		BR	120-150	121	TL	150-225
91	TL	100-125	106	TL	150-200		TR	1200-1500
	TR	75-100		TR	125-175	122	CL	25-50
	CL	40-60		BR	175-225		TR	75-150
		50-75	107	TL	150-200			30-75
	CR	35-50		TR	100-150		BL	100-150
	BL	50-75		BL	275-400	124	TR	40-60
92	TL	65-85	108	TR	110-180		CL	50-75
		75-100		BR	100-150		CR	30-50
	CL	60-75			100-140		BL	75-100
		60-75	109	TL	150-200		BR	80-100
	BC	30-50		TR	125-200	125	TL	40-60
93	TR	40-50		BL	125-200		CR	40-60
	BL	85-100		BR	125-200		BR	75-150
94	TL	60-80			125-200	126	TL	100-125
	TR	50-75	110	TR	110-180		TR	25-50
	BR	12-18		BL	120-180		BL	100-125
95	TL	40-50		BR	100-175		BR	10-25
96	TR	50-70	111	TL	90-150	127		10-50
	BR	25-30		BL	90-120	129	TL	35-50
97	CL	40-50	112	CL	140-160		TR	40-55
	TR	50-75		TR	125-200		CL	50-65
	CR	125-150		BL	125-200		CR	50-60
	BR	75-100			125-200	132	CR	60-75
98	TR	50-60	113	CL	120-200		BL	100-150
	CL	60-75		TR	125-200		BR	70-85
	BR	90-110		BR	125-200	133	TL	50-75
99	BR	60-100	114	BR	250-325			50-75
100	TL	60-100	115	C & BL	200-275		TR	200-250
	TR	75-100		T & CR	450-600		CL	50-65
	CL	60-100			400-450		BR	55-95

No.	Pos.	Value	No.	Pos.	Value	No.	Pos.	Value
134	CR	150-170		BL	65-85		TR	30-90
		(in orig. cond.)		BR	60-75		BR	35-80
	CL	65-110	145	TR	125-175	157	TL & R	35-125
	BL	50-75		BL	125-150		BL	35-80
		75-100		BR	100-125	158	TL	10-15
		50-75	146	TL	75-125		TR	40-90
135	TL	40-60			75-125		BR	40-60/ea.
	TR	80-100/set		TR	75-125	159	TL	80-120
	CL	125-150			75-125		TR	100-125
	CR	75-100		BL	80-130		BL	75-100
		75-100			100-150		BR	30-75
	BC	75-125	147	TL	75-100	160	TL	175-225
136		225-275		TR	75-90			40-60
137	TC	75-125		BR	35-50		TR	60-75
	C	30-40			40-60		BR	30-40
		40-50			70-90	161	T&BL	75-125
	BC	25-50	148	TR	150-175		CR	75-100
138	TL	70-90			300-350	163	CR	20-25
	TR	50-150		CL	400-700	164	TR	20-40/ea.
	BL	70-90		CR	225-275		BL	10-15
	BR	100-125			50-65	168	CR	30-40
		75-90		BL	550-650			15-30/ea.
139	TL	40-50	149	CL	325-400	169	TL	60-130
	CR	20-30		R	350-400			40-80
	BR	225-275			250-300		BR	45-60
140	TR	35-65			800-900			25-40
	CR	200-250			250-275	175	TR	40-60
	BR	150-175			190-225		CR	10-15
141	TL	1,00-1,100			200-250		BR	70-100
		95-125		BC	200-225	176	TL	30-40
	CR	150-200	150	TR	150-175		BL	150-200
	BL	300-350		BL	90-125	177	TL	25-35
		225-275	151	TR	20-50		BR	25-50
142	TL	150-200		BR	20-75	178	BR	75-100
	CR	60-80	152	CR	20-50/ea.			(excluding cap and apron)
		60-80		BR	20-60/ea.	180	BL	25-35
143	TL	40-60	153	TL	20-60/ea.	184	BL	25-35
		60-80		TR	25-75		CR	100-125
		40-60		BL	10-25			
	TR	40-60	154	TL	25-40	185	TL	100-115
		20-30		TR	100-140		CL	100-115
	BL	60-80		BL	40-60		BR	75-100
		25-50		BR	50-75	186	TL	25-30
144	TL	60-75	155	BR	140-250		CL	20-45
	TR	80-100	156	TL	75-135		BR	40-50

INDEX